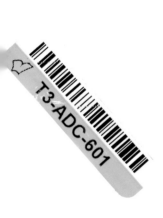

ExTension

The 20-Minute-a-Day Yoga-Based Program
to Relax, Release, and Rejuvenate
the Average Stressed-Out Over-35-Year-Old Body

SAM DWORKIS

with Peg Moline

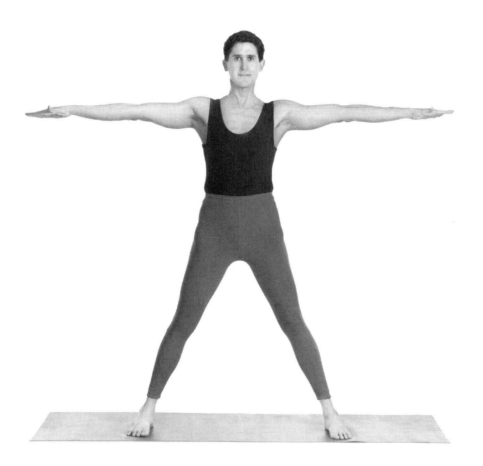

Photographs by Ellen Wallop   Design by Chik Shank

POSEIDON PRESS

New York   London   Toronto   Sydney   Tokyo   Singapore

POSEIDON PRESS
Rockefeller Center
1230 Avenue of the Americas
New York, New York 10020

POSEIDON PRESS is a registered trademark of Simon & Schuster Inc.
POSEIDON PRESS colophon is a trademark of Simon & Schuster Inc.

Designed by Shank Design

Manufactured in the United States of America

1 3 5 7 9 10 8 6 4 2

Library of Congress Cataloging-in-Publication Data
Dworkis, Sam
ExTension: the 20-minute-a-day, yoga-based program to relax, release, and
rejuvenate the average stressed-out over-35-year-old body / Sam Dworkis with Peg Moline.
p.   cm.
1. Yoga, Hatha — Therapeutic use.   2. Middle aged persons — Health and hygiene. I. Moline, Peg. II. Title.
RA 781.7.D88   1994
613.7'046—dc20   93-41908
CIP

ISBN: 0-671-86680-X

Bachin Charts: "The Muscular System" and "The Skeletal System."
Courtesy of Anatomy Chart Company, Skokie, Illinois. Used with permission.

Fascia photos from C. D. Clemente, *Anatomy. A Regional Atlas of the Human Body*, 3d ed.
(Philadelphia; Lea & Febiger/Munich, Urban & Schwarzenburg, 1987). Used with permission.

The techniques, ideas, and suggestions in this book are not intended as a substitute
for proper medical advice. Consult your physician or health care professional before beginning
this or any new exercise program, particularly if you are pregnant or nursing, or if you are elderly
or if you have any chronic or recurring physical conditions. Any application of the techniques,
ideas, and suggestions in this book is at the reader's sole discretion and risk.

TO JANE

Without your love, encouragement, and help...
this book could not have been possible.

ACKNOWLEDGMENTS

I wish to thank all my teachers, students, and colleagues who have given me much more than time. They have given me inspiration. I specifically wish to thank Mr. BKS Iyengar, whose knowledge and understanding of yoga have profoundly influenced me and thousands of others throughout the world; Jerry Bird, who first encouraged me to teach; Bobbi Goldin and Susan Virant, both of whom encouraged me further to explore my personal and professional potential; Paul St. John and Judith Walker, who encouraged excellence in understanding human anatomy and function; Peg Moline, who helped organize my teaching, thoughts, and experience into the written word; Ellen Wallop, New York sports and fitness photographer, who was able to capture my teaching and concepts on film; my longtime friends Chik and Laurie Shank of Shank Design, Miami, whose brilliance in design and Macintosh publishing are evident throughout these pages; Wilbert van den Braak, who provided me a "MacOffice" so that I could complete my manuscript; my models, MJ Salk, Annie Jubb, and, of course, Susan Virant, who was willing to go beyond expectations to complete the photographs; Don Cleary, who, having eliminated his back pain through ExTension, has become my agent and friend, always there to offer invaluable assistance and insight; and finally, my publisher and student, Ann Patty, who believed in ExTension from the beginning.

Whatever you may think of yoga, whatever stories you may have heard, whatever strange things you may suspect — think again! Sam Dworkis has created a new approach to yoga that is for everyone. Yoga — thousands of years old — is one of the most valuable physical disciplines known to us. Sam's system bridges the gap between fitness and wellness, from Eastern thought to Western logic.

After years of lying around and eating fast food, or, on the other hand, doing traditional Western fitness to excess, we may all be in dire need of this very effective yoga system. Personally, I've done the latter (though I must admit I've done my share of lying around), and after twelve years of teaching classes, doing videos, and leading workshops for aerobics instructors, I am pooped! I've been through all the fitness programs of the nineties: high impact, low impact, circuit, interval, step — you name it, I've overdone it! I certainly needed to slow down. Rethink. Chill out.

Enter yoga. I had been studying yoga for about one year when I met Sam and he introduced me to his ExTension system of yoga. Finally, a system that includes everyone — my mom can do it and can even relate to it. I certainly warmed up to the idea that less is more, and by actually doing less I had more energy! But even if you usually don't overdo, don't worry — you can handle it. It's manageable yet effective.

Remember, as we get older we begin to lose strength and flexibility. Sam's program helps soften the aging process yet harden the body in all the right spots to keep you healthy. Yoga also relieves stress, increases oxygen capacity, helps with mental clarity, and just gives you a great sense of peace.

I personally look forward to this new swing in fitness. Balanced, gentle yet effective, safe, and harmonious in spirit. Go for it! Give it a good honest try! See if you don't just feel and look better and, of course, have more time and energy to enjoy your life. Now, that's a great reason to exercise.

May you enjoy Sam's program as much as I have, and may your life be full and your spirit free.

Molly Fox

CONTENTS

CONTENTS

CONTENTS

PART III

ExTension Is for You If:

1. You're stressed out. Or feeling out of shape. Or eating too much. You feel it's time for a change but can't seem to get started. Maybe you have no idea where to begin.

2. You're over...a certain age. Let's say over 35. You feel young, but your body keeps letting you down.

3. You know exercise is good for you, but you've given up on it because
    - you've tried exercise classes and programs but they don't deliver what they promise.
    - you feel so far out of shape that you can't get back.
    - you feel too "old" or feel frustrated because most exercise programs are too difficult for you.
    - you can't find the time.
    - you can't do the exercise and sports you used to do well.
    - you're injured or seem to get hurt frequently.
    - you have a bad back or bad knees.
    - you feel too tired, fatigued, or sore.
    - equipment, classes, or health club memberships cost too much.

4. You're an athlete, dancer, or "weekend athlete" who wants to
    - improve performance through enhanced flexibility and strength training.
    - prevent injuries by stretching and strengthening.
    - stay in shape while minor injuries heal.

5. You're an athlete or dancer who wants to stop abusing your body.

6. You love to exercise but want to try something different.

7. You've thought about yoga but you think you're not flexible enough or yoga is too weird.

8. You already practice yoga, keep getting injured, or are looking for a different way that may serve you better.

9. YOU WANT TO FEEL GOOD AGAIN.

Part I

ExTension

Introducing a Program That Works

Yoga for the Western Body

Are you just plain tired of your body sometimes? And so stressed out you can't even think about relaxing? You know that exercise would probably make you feel better, but it seems too hard, takes too much time, or just doesn't seem to work. You can't seem to stick with it for any length of time. You try and try, get sore, injured, or discouraged, and then you quit. Why can't you exercise the way you want to or the way you used to? What changed?

As hard as it is to accept, you have changed. As you get older your body changes, too. But that doesn't mean you have to give up exercise. In fact, it's more important than ever. It does mean that you need to understand what's happening to your body and what you can do about it.

That's what this book is all about. It's an easy-to-learn exercise program that fits into your life. Once you learn it, it takes very little time — just 20 minutes a day, four to six days a week — virtually no equipment and hardly any space. And it works.

The program is called ExTension. It's based on a system — yoga — that has been around for centuries; you could say that it's the most successful exercise trend of all time. The ExTension program will not only increase your flexibility, it will improve your posture, flatten your belly, and firm your arms and thighs. It will release tension and reduce stress. Once you learn it, you can do it as an aerobic exercise to burn fat. It will get you moving. Or you can do it slowly as "meditation in action." It will relax you. It will keep you looking and feeling young.

ExTension is based on yoga exercise because I believe it's a nearly perfect form of exercise. It enhances every facet of physical and emotional fitness: strength, endurance, flexibility, posture, balance, stress management, and concentration. But traditional yoga had to be adapted to be better suited for the Western body and mind. It had to be made easy and unintimidating to people afraid to try it. And it had to be adapted to work for those of us moving into our 40s and 50s.

Yoga can also help you to maintain a healthy, pain-free body. In a survey for their book *Backache Relief* (hardback: New York: Times Books/Random House, 1985; paperback: New York: NAL/Signet Books, 1986) Arthur Klein and Dava Sobel asked 492 chronic back-pain sufferers what provided them with the most dramatic long-term relief, and 96 percent said "yoga" more than chiropractic, physical therapy, or surgery (see the survey results in Appendix V).

Executives around the country are using yoga for exercise and for stress reduction. Pro basketball star Kareem Abdul-Jabbar, the highest-scoring and — before he retired — the oldest player in the history of the game, credits yoga exercise for his long, injury-free career. And yoga exercise is gaining new popularity with regular folks who appreciate the suppleness, the vitality, and the energy it gives them.

The problem is that most people won't try yoga. They don't have the time to go to a class several times a week. They think they're too stiff or that it's too hard. They imagine yoga students twisting themselves into pretzel shapes and chanting in smoky, candle-lit rooms. Most classical forms of yoga can be intimidating and difficult to learn and especially difficult to learn from a book. That's why I developed ExTension.

ExTension makes yoga, that most perfect form of exercise, *easy*. And it doesn't matter how flexible or stiff, young or old, you are.

How to Use This Book

If you're anything like me, you'll want to jump right into the exercise program and skip the introduction and tests.

Don't. Read the book first.

And do all the tests and "proofs" as you read them. (A proof is a test that shows you — physically — why something I'm teaching you works. They're actually pretty fun, and you'll learn a lot about yourself.)

It sounds simple, but the entire ExTension program is based on setting down firm foundations for your body and understanding the principles on which it's based. If you take time now to read and learn these foundations, when you actually start working, things will happen very quickly, and the results you get will last. Otherwise, this becomes just another exercise program that you'll try for a while and then quit because it won't make sense to you or it won't live up to your expectations.

As you continue to read and use this book, you'll uncover layers and layers of information. The more you practice it and read the details, the more they (and the whole ExTension program) will mean to you. The first time you try it, you'll get some of the details; the next time, things that weren't clear at first will begin to make sense. So don't worry if you don't get everything right away. Just keep doing it; the details will evolve and you'll find yourself going deeper and deeper into it.

Also, as you start getting into the program and understanding these details, you'll move through your day better. When you bend down to get a can off the bottom shelf, for example, or twist around for something in the backseat of your car, you'll do it differently.

Part I defines the foundations and principles and teaches you how to apply them to the actual ExTension program in Part II. You will then be able to practice the program safely.

In Part I you'll also find a series of physical and personality tests that will let you make this your own customized program. Take them, make note of the results, then go to Part II.

Part II is the heart of the book — the exercises. And this is when you will start training your body and learning how to practice.

Be sure to read Part III. This section gives you a deeper understanding of ExTension that will enhance your practice. You will be able to increase your benefits while spending less time doing it.

Finally, the Appendixes offer you some variations and additional information that tests traditional ways of doing selected exercises so that there will be absolutely no doubt in your mind that ExTension works.

Throughout the book, you'll see boxes and sections:

Body Types: This program acknowledges that everyone has different degrees of flexibility. Therefore, the exercises are adapted for Tight, Moderate, and Flexible body types. You'll find out which you are in "Know Your Body" in Part I. This section tells you — in general terms — which examples to follow.

Attitude Adjustments: You'll also be assessing your personality, figuring out your approach to exercise and life, and coming up with an evaluation as to whether you are Aggressive, Moderate, or Easygoing. Some, not all, of the exercises will have instructions for your personality type to help you get even more from the exercises and keep you from getting hurt by pushing yourself too hard.

Cautions: These are special instructions. Some are warnings for people with preexisting conditions such as high blood pressure, heart disease, or back problems. Some are simply preparations for the exercises.

What You'll Feel: What you look like while you do these exercises is not as important as how you feel while doing them. The material in these boxes tells you what you can expect to feel if you're doing the movements correctly for your body type.

Fine-Tuning: This is just what it says, a way to fine-tune the movement once you get the basics down. ExTension is a program with many levels and details. Each time you go through the program, you'll learn more and more. Something you didn't quite get yesterday will become crystal clear today. A detail that evaded your body during week one will suddenly click during week two. That's why this program will never get stale. Fine-Tuning will keep you on your toes.

The "Nix" Sign: Next to selected photographs, you'll see the nix sign. This means that the photograph depicts a wrong or dangerous way to do an exercise. Try it if you wish so that you can compare it with the correct method. But remember to go slowly and avoid pushing into pain.

THE HISTORY BEHIND EXTENSION

Before I started doing yoga some 18 years ago, I was 30, a banker, in graduate school, playing a lot of basketball and running. I was becoming so stiff that it was getting in the way of practically everything I did. I had heard about yoga. I knew some people who practiced it, but I had no inclination to do something so passive. Like so many other people, I was afraid that I was not inherently flexible enough and I certainly had no desire to practice an Eastern religion.

Then I met a man on the basketball court who moved differently from anyone I had ever played against. His attitude was different too. It's not that he was laid back, but he seemed to play better under pressure than the other guys. I asked him about it. He told me that he had been doing yoga and that it changed his game. He was right. It almost immediately changed my game. And, ultimately, my life.

But not at first. I approached the yoga exercises with the same aggressive zeal that I approached my other exercises. I couldn't understand why, if yoga was supposed to be so good for you, I kept getting injured — a muscle pain here, a muscle strain there. A knee injury. A back injury.

Through the years, I noticed that only the most flexible people found yoga easy and enjoyable. Almost all students over 40 and especially the stiffer people had a hard time, and most of them dropped out after the first couple of classes. But those who persisted, as I did, experienced injuries. Even many of the flexible people were getting injured. Especially when they pushed their postures or tried to progress too quickly. Many of them ultimately developed neck, spine and joint problems.

Overall, I liked how I was feeling about my body. But I couldn't understand why so many people were getting hurt and why so many people were dropping out. I knew that yoga was beneficial. We just weren't practicing it right. So I decided to study with the masters. I went to Europe and India several times to study with the world's best instructors. But I still didn't learn why it seemed so difficult for those of us approaching middle age or older and why I kept getting hurt.

About eight years ago, I began studying NeuroMuscular therapy. Applying those physiological principles to my yoga practice changed everything. I began to understand HOW and WHY yoga works and why we get injured when we do the postures wrong. I learned how our bodies change as we grow older, as we pass from our 30s to the 40s, 50s, and beyond. I discovered why exercise becomes more difficult as we pass through these ten-year thresholds. As I modified my personal practice and teaching, I not only felt better in my body but also realized that my students of all ages and physical conditions were able to learn much more quickly than before, with much quicker results, and, most important, without injury.

Yoga exercise is one of the best kinds of exercise you can do. It helps you to feel and look young, strong, and beautiful.

And that's why I began to develop ExTension based on yoga exercises but also on solid, proven physiological principles; not on tradition, belief, opinion, or philosophy.

ExTension is the result of 17 years of passionate research, practice, and lots of trial and error. With it, I want to teach you why yoga exercise works, why your body changes as you age, why exercise may not feel as good as it used to, and how to do an exercise program — ExTension — that will change your life. As you begin to understand why certain exercises work (and why others don't), you'll also begin to enjoy the movement and the new vitality you feel. If you simply follow the leader in classes, books, or tapes, you may not understand what you're doing. You may struggle, become bored or injured, and stop altogether. Sound familiar?

The term "ExTension" comes from one of the physiological principles on which the program is based: ExTension releases tension. It has a double meaning. By extending through the muscles of your arms, legs, spine, and even your fingers, you get rid of the tension and imbalance that can build up as you do the exercises. (In yoga, they are called postures, or poses.) The exercises become more effective, and they feel better as you do them.

And the subtitle of this book, "Relax, release, and rejuvenate," is a promise I intend to keep. Get into this practice and you'll naturally feel relaxed both after your exercise session and during your day; you'll release physical and mental tension, and you'll live life with an incredible well of energy.

But before you get started, learn the principles that form the foundation of this program, starting with a quick anatomy lesson. If you'd like more detail, refer to Appendix I. I promise, if you follow the instructions and do it correctly, this won't hurt a bit.

It's hard to boil down years of experience and study into a few statements and sometimes even harder to read those statements. But the key to this program is the details, and you need to understand why ExTension works, why it feels better, and why the program is one you can do for the rest of your life.

In this program, we're interested in four types of soft tissue: muscle, tendon, ligament, and, above all, fascia. Basically, muscles move our bodies; they are infused with blood and, when they're injured, heal pretty quickly. Tendons attach muscle to bone; they contain very little blood and take longer to heal. Ligament connects bone to bone and has almost no blood circulation. A ligament injury almost certainly means surgery.

Covering your entire body is a fourth connective tissue, called fascia. When you pull the skin off a chicken breast, you find a whitish fiber between the meat and skin. That's fascia, and you have it, too. It not only covers your body, it permeates every muscle fiber and all your organs and glands.

As you go through life, you inevitably injure yourself, either through accidents or simple wear and tear. You heal, but the muscles, tendons, ligament, and fascia of your body "remember" the injury. Especially the fascia. About every ten years — ages 28 to 32, 38 to 42, 48 to 52, 58 to 62 and 68 to 72 — your fascia becomes less resilient, and those past injuries cause it to become tighter and tighter. As your fascia becomes contracted, other parts of your body suffer. And if other parts of your body suffer, your fascia contracts even more.

Even the simple act of trying to remain upright every day becomes a fatiguing chore. If your body is out of alignment, your muscles constantly contract to keep you standing or sitting. Your fascia contracts with them, and by nightfall you feel as though you've been carrying around the world.

ExTension works to release fascia. It works on the surface level and gently, layer by layer, relaxes and releases tight fascia…and you begin to feel rejuvenated.

Most exercise, including most other yoga systems, goes too deep too quickly, flexes the joints and spine too much, and sets up a chain reaction of irritation and pain within the muscles and fascia.

Translation? If it hurts deeply, don't do it. Lighten up, and you'll open up that fascia, and the rest of your soft tissue will respond. There really is no gain in pain. The proof is in Hilton's Law of soft tissue.

PRINCIPLE # 1: HILTON'S LAW

In the late 1800s, a scientist named John Hilton postulated that the nerve root that supplies a joint supplies all the muscles, ligaments, and tendons that attach to that joint, as well the overlying skin. And if Hilton's Law (taken from *Dorland's Illustrated Medical Dictionary*) is correct, that means the nerve root must also travel through the fascia surrounding the muscles and underneath the skin. If a joint, say your elbow, is injured, the nerve sends a message to all the surrounding tissues — muscles, skin, fascia — telling them to contract; it's the body's way of immobilizing the tissue so it can heal. At the same time, your nervous system is under extreme stimulation from the injury; the more stimulated your nervous system, the more general contraction takes place. It becomes a nasty downward spiral. That is why you have to avoid pain and keep your stretching confined to areas filled with thick, healthy muscle tissue.

If you've ever had surgery, you've experienced Hilton's Law; it feels as if every muscle in your body is contracted. Hilton's Law is the key to the ExTension system.

PRINCIPLE #2: PAIN

Pain is a message that something is wrong and needs to be changed. Or stopped. If you're performing a movement or holding a position that hurts, you must find a way to do it differently or stop doing it altogether. Otherwise, you'll inhibit your progress by setting up a chain reaction of irritation and pain. Pain in your neck, back, knees, or the sitting bones in your buttocks is especially crucial to avoid. Never push into pain in those areas.

The message in the pain may be "Stop!" When an animal is injured, it doesn't get up and try to continue its life. It finds a dark place to hide and lies down until it heals. Sometimes you just have to stop and maybe lie down.

PRINCIPLE #3: LESS GETS YOU MORE

All your life — and especially during the fitness-crazed years — you've been told that good things have to be hard to get. If there's no pain, there's no gain. Fortunately, in this decade, we've gotten smarter, and we're getting away from that dangerous thinking. But it's still tough to believe that if a little is good, more isn't necessarily better.

You're going to learn, however, that within the ExTension program, less is more. Once you learn how to move with proper alignment, extending your body without hurting your muscles, tendons, fascia, or joints, less will always get you more. This means less aggression, less effort, and less pain; more flexibility, strength, endurance, and tone.

PRINCIPLE #4: PROPER STRETCHING

Any time you create an action (a stretch, a feeling that something is happening) close to or in a joint, you are stretching tendon or ligament. It is safer (and more productive) to create action first in muscle (such as the hamstrings). Then, as the muscle relaxes and begins to stretch, you can take the action closer to the joint (toward the tendon) but never deep into the joint (ligament).

PRINCIPLE #5: EXTENSION RELEASES TENSION

Any exercise program will improve how you feel, even if you move lazily through it. But if you extend your neck, limbs, spine, and fingers long as you exercise, the movements will feel better and work better. Extension through your joints creates freedom of movement; compression restricts movement. This applies to all of your joints, including your knees, elbows, hips, and, especially, your spine. When you elongate through your joints, pain is reduced and you feel lighter. Compressing into your joints creates pain and you feel heavier.

Test this out. Lie down on your back, legs flat on the floor. Now lift your right leg and hold it about six to nine inches off the floor [Figs.1 and 2]. Just hold it up. Notice how it feels. Does it become heavy or start to shake? It will probably become pretty uncomfortable as you keep holding it up. Put the leg back down and rest.

Now, you will learn how to create an "active" leg. Point your left heel away from you while you push through the ball of your foot and stretch your entire leg out away from you. Continue holding your leg up as you extend it long [Figs. 3 and 4]. Notice how much lighter your leg feels.

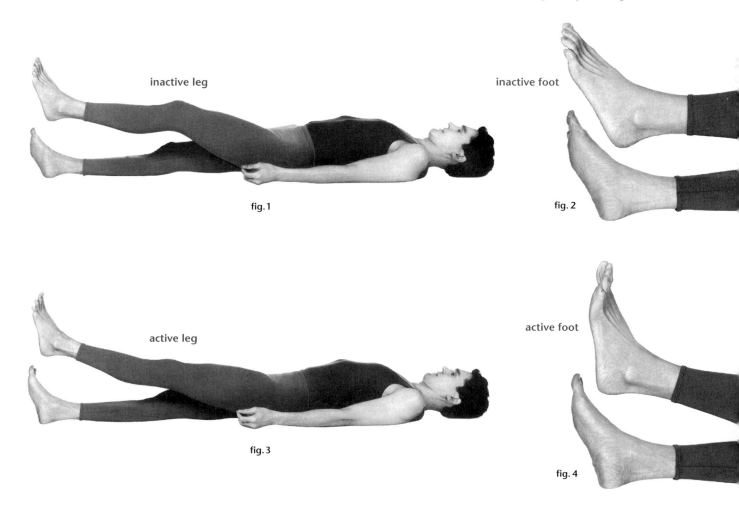

inactive leg

fig.1

inactive foot

fig. 2

active leg

fig.3

active foot

fig. 4

Now for a moment, completely relax the foot and leg while you are holding it up. It becomes heavy again. Extend it once more. Lighter. Lower your leg and test this process with your left leg.

The extension you created released the tension of holding up your leg. It works with your arms, your spine, your head, and your neck. It will make any exercise you do feel and work better. EXTENSION RELEASES TENSION. You'll see this phrase again and again in this book. It has become a sort of mantra for my students. See Appendix I for a further discussion of this principle.

PRINCIPLE #6: LENGTHENING THE SPINE INCREASES ACTION

In this book, you're going to be told (often) to lengthen your spine. You might be standing, sitting, or lying down. All it means is to think yourself longer, from your tailbone to the top of your head. But this action serves a very important purpose, and it goes back to Principle #5: ExTension releases tension. Lengthening your spine lets you breathe more freely, it enhances the stretch you feel, and it helps your circulation and digestion. If you compress your spine, or slump, these processes become restricted.

PRINCIPLE #7: THE IMPORTANCE OF BREATH

Deep, smooth, rhythmic breathing makes exercise easier and more effective than shallow breathing or holding your breath.

You can live without food for about 30 days; without water for about three to six. But you can survive without oxygen for only four to six minutes before you start to suffocate. Obviously, breath is very important to the sustenance of life. But breath also has a profound effect on your body during exercise and on your nervous system.

I'm sure you've been in a pressure situation and realized you were holding your breath. If you stopped to think about it, it was hard to think, hard to move or do anything, really. What you will discover is that if you don't hold your breath, if you allow your exhalation and inhalation to flow freely, these exercises will feel much more comfortable and powerful. Not only are you allowing the breath to do its job of flushing and replenishing the muscles, but the rush of air into and out of your nose stimulates a relaxation response in your nervous system. That's one reason we strive to breathe through the nose; it also warms and filters the air.

If you find nasal breathing uncomfortable, simply breathe through your mouth. With this practice, most "mouth breathers" are soon able to breathe comfortably through the nose. Remember; anything that restricts your breath works against you.

PRINCIPLE #8: ACTIVE RELAXATION

I participated in a research project at Wright Patterson Air Force Base that observed brain function during rest, exercise, task orientation (physical and mental coordination exercises), and yoga. The researchers, among other things, wanted to see if an alpha state (deep mental relaxation and quietness) could be generated in the brain during exercise. Alpha is generated when the body is quiet and relaxed, sitting or lying down with the eyes closed.

We postulated that if you could place your body in a perfectly balanced position, and maintain that balance while you move, your body would release tension and your brain would generate alpha, even while you exercise.

Creating that balance means activating your entire body, that is, using the "extension releases tension" principle equally for your hands and arms, feet and legs, spine and neck. Maintaining an equal feeling of extension throughout your body while you move. If, for example, you extend your hands but keep your legs soft, there is imbalance within your body, and your brain must remain active to keep you from falling over.

We found that you can go into a moving alpha state (even with your eyes open!) by creating that balanced state of extension in all the muscles of your body and by breathing deeply and easily. In fact, you can be meditating while you exercise.

You'll be learning an exercise, the Arm Flap, as part of a sequence called Sun Salutations. In it, you'll experience the balance of your body during movement. You'll learn how to put together everything I've been hinting at: extending your muscles; widening your shoulders; how to activate your hands, fingers together, thumbs stretching away; elbows stretching away from shoulders; kneecaps lifting up; spine lengthening; lungs expanding. You'll learn how to bring on a state of active rest, of energetic relaxation. That's what yoga teaches you.

CAUTION

**Do not hold your breath during these exercises.
You will be unable to maximize the benefits available to you.**

TEST YOUR FLEXIBILITY AND YOUR PERSONALITY

You are an individual. And as an individual, you're probably frustrated by trying to follow an exercise program designed for everybody else or by trying to participate in a class in which you're just another number.

In the ExTension program, I ask you not to follow blindly what I — or any other exercise instructor — tell you to do, not to forge ahead without knowing what you're doing or why. The problem with most exercise classes is that everyone is trying to copy the teacher. I don't want you to try to look like me or anyone else while you're doing these exercises.

The reason I want you to test your flexibility before you start is that many of the elements of this program have been developed through the practice and study of yoga. To follow the exercises safely, and not try to look like one perfect example, you need some guidelines so you can work within the limits of your current flexibility.

And that flexibility doesn't have to be great. Yoga means union, or balance. This means a balance between strength, endurance, and flexibility. I believe that people who are very flexible, yet lack a balance of requisite strength, are imbalanced in their musculature. And my goal with this book is to help you enhance, not just your flexibility, but your strength and endurance as well.

ExTension will work only if you realistically recognize your current level of strength and flexibility. Not what it was ten years ago, or what you wish it were. So the first step is to assess your body through the following tests. The second is to evaluate your attitude toward exercise and life in general.

ASSESS YOUR FLEXIBILITY

The following tests will help you assess your general flexibility in the back of your body, mainly your hamstrings and back muscles; and your upper body, mainly your chest and shoulder muscles. Take the tests as directed, but remember, this isn't a contest. Don't judge yourself, and above all, don't hurt yourself.

For each test you'll type yourself Tight, Moderate, or Flexible. When you finish with the tests, you'll have an idea both of your overall flexibility and of your flexibility in specific body areas for specific exercises. You may actually be flexible in one area of your body and tight in another. You'll also have some general guidelines for doing the exercises in Part II.

Each exercise in this book is demonstrated (with equal importance) for the Tight, Moderate, and Flexible body types. You'll even see some Very Tight examples. The tests you're about to take will tell you which example you should follow as you learn each exercise, but please remember three things:

1. The reason you need to type yourself — physically and mentally — is so that you will be doing your exercise, not someone else's. For example, don't be tempted to make yourself look flexible or to try the Flexible example if, in fact, your body is generally tight by pushing yourself into an exercise. I call this "aggression." It will get you nowhere. In fact, aggressiveness will ultimately impede your progress. Even if you've successfully pushed hard all your life and have been rewarded for your efforts, in this program, pushing yourself into an exercise that is inappropriate for your body type might discourage you, or worse, it may hurt you. These are two reasons you may not be exercising in the first place. So don't do it. Don't pay attention to anyone's body but your own.

2. When you're beginning the program (and especially if you've never done yoga exercise before) I recommend testing out the Tight example first. If the correct form comes easily to you, then progress to the Moderate or Flexible position.

3. People have varying degrees of flexibility in different parts of their bodies. When you begin the exercise program you may find, for example, that you're a Tight body type in a particular exercise, a Moderate in another exercise, and a Flexible in still another. That's why you need to test and learn your own physical ability within each exercise and not just follow one body type throughout. It's also why you'll see our models demonstrating the Tight adaptation for one particular exercise and the Flexible example for another.

You could even be Moderate on one day and Tight on another day. How much movement you have, and how the exercises feel, on any given day is what's important. Read the directions for each exercise carefully, paying particular attention to the descriptions of what you may expect to experience while you're doing them. This is the key to reducing your stress and to improving your stamina, strength, and flexibility.

While you're doing these tests, also notice your level of internal tension or frustration. You'll use that for the personality tests later on.

FINE-TUNING

Always read ahead first before you proceed with an actual test or exercise so that you'll know what to expect.

The Lying Down Hamstring Stretch Test

This hamstring stretch, done lying down on your back, is a good measure of the flexibility of the muscles in the back of your legs. It slightly duplicates the Standing Hamstring Stretch that follows, but it's somewhat easier and definitely safer to feel a hamstring stretch while on your back. More important, though, it lets you test each leg separately; you may find that you're more flexible in one leg than the other.

The hamstring stretch is also a very important component of this program; you'll learn more about it as you read on.

CAUTION

You must keep your thigh touching or at least moving toward your chest throughout this test. Be sure to keep your tailbone down on the floor. And as always, remember to breathe deeply.

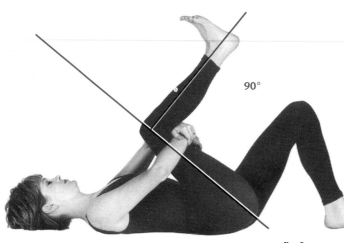

90°

fig. 5

Lie next to a mirror on your back, with your knees bent, feet flat on the floor. Keeping your left foot down, bend your right knee and bring it toward your chest. Wrap your arms underneath your thigh, then hold on to your hands, wrists, or elbows. If you can't reach around your thigh at all, put a towel around it and hold both ends.

Now, inhale, dorsiflex your foot (that's extending your heel away from you), and gently pull your thigh toward your chest, keeping your knees bent. When you've brought your thigh as close to your chest as you can *and are holding it in place*, slowly unbend your knee, while you are exhaling, as far as you comfortably can. Stop when you feel a stretch — not a pain — in your hamstrings or when you run out of exhalation.

Look at yourself in the mirror, then compare your hamstring stretch to those here. After making sure your tailbone is firmly down on the floor, the first thing to look at in each of these examples is the angle of the shin to the thigh.

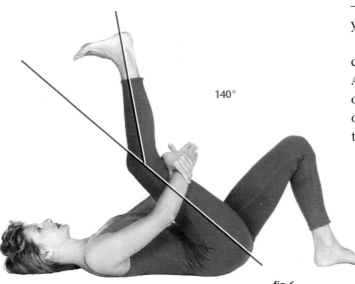

140°

fig. 6

▶ Tight

MJ can bring her thigh reasonably close to her chest although she can barely hold both wrists [Fig. 5]. When she unbends her knee, her ankle to her thigh forms just about a right angle. If you can unbend your leg about 90 degrees or less, your flexibility is Tight for this test.

▶ Moderate

Susan gets her thigh just a little closer to her chest than MJ [Fig. 6]. But look how much more she can straighten her leg, allowing her to grasp both wrists easily. Her knee forms about a 120-degree angle. If your hamstring stretch looks like Susan's, your flexibility is Moderate.

▶ Flexible

I am demonstrating the most flexible position [Fig. 7]. My thigh nearly rests on my chest, and I am able to unbend my knee about 135 degrees. I easily hold on to both elbows. If your hamstring stretch comes close to this, consider yourself Flexible here.

WHAT YOU'LL FEEL

If you feel any pain or tightness behind your knee (or anywhere in your leg), you have pushed too far. The stretch should be centered midway between the back of your knee and the sitting bone in your buttock; in other words, in the "belly" of your hamstrings. At this point, it is important that you know the difference between muscle, tendon, and ligament. If you don't, please refer now to "Why ExTension Works" in Appendix I.

IF YOU CAN'T FEEL A STRETCH WHEN YOU DO THIS TEST

The hamstring stretch, centered in the belly of your muscle, is the core of this program. I want you to be able to feel it there, not behind your knees or in your back.

Some of you will be tempted to move ahead before you really know what this means and before you feel this stretch in the right place.

*I appreciate your enthusiasm but I encourage you to go slowly enough to feel and really isolate the stretch in your hamstrings. Take the time now. If you do, this program will work extremely well for you. But if you plow ahead without isolating an accurate stretch in your hamstrings, you won't be able to get the most from this program, and, more than likely, **you will irritate your back and quit.** If you can't feel a hamstring stretch in this or in the standing hamstring test, it could be because you're either too flexible or too tight. Turn now to Appendix III, "Variation for Hamstring Stretching." Practice this variation for as long as it takes before you continue with the ExTension program, or you won't get anywhere with it. It might take you several minutes or it might you take several days, but you must be able to feel clearly an isolated stretch in your hamstrings before you proceed. Don't quit. You will do it, and then you can safely continue on with the next step.*

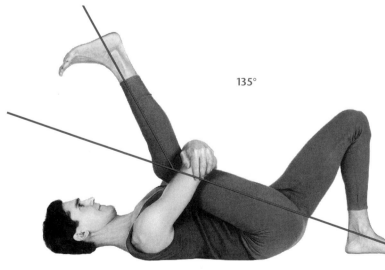

135°

fig. 7

Arms Overhead Test

The flexibility of your chest, upper back, neck, and shoulders is an important (and often overlooked) factor in exercise.
If you do an exercise that tightens up any part of your shoulders — top, behind your neck, or behind your shoulder blades — you can't help tensing your neck, which ultimately restricts your breathing as well. Also, tight muscles of the neck and shoulders can give you headaches.

The Arms Overhead test checks the flexibility of your chest and shoulders and teaches you a different way to raise your arms without creating tension in your neck. It will tell you which example you'll probably follow when you do the Arm Flap, Cobra, and Downward Facing Dog exercises to come.

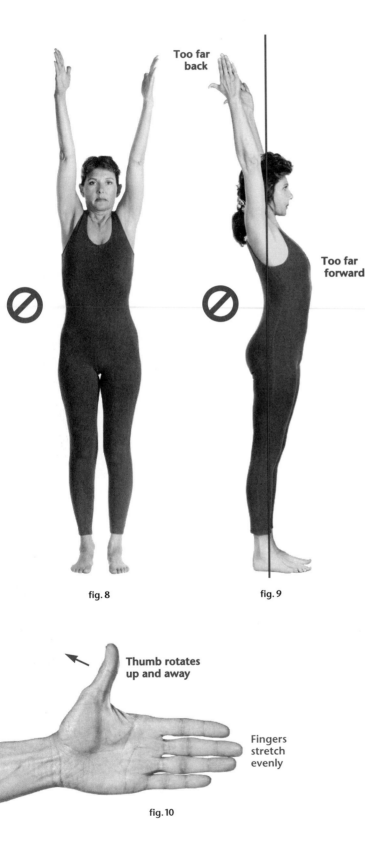

Too far
back

Too far
forward

fig. 8   fig. 9

Thumb rotates
up and away

Fingers
stretch
evenly

fig. 10

Stand facing a mirror and simply stretch your arms up and over your head. How does it feel? Do you feel any tightness in your neck and shoulders? How does it look? Compare your posture to Susan's in Figure 8. Now turn sideways and notice what's happening to the back of your shoulders. Are they hunching up too? Are you bringing your arms too far behind you, which throws your chest forward and overarches your lower back? (Susan demonstrates this in Figure 9.) Take your arms back down and face the mirror.

Before you raise your arms the second time, take a breath, and as you exhale and lift your arms up sideways, consciously bring your shoulders down and wide. Think about increasing the space between your shoulder blades and between the ends of your collarbones. Imagine the muscles below your armpits (your lats) pulling away from the sides of your back. Bring the fingers of each hand together, extend them long, and pull your thumb away from the rest of your fingers. It's called activating your hands; you'll be doing a lot of it in ExTension [Fig. 10, active hand detail].

Hold on to that feeling of widening the shoulders — you'll be using this several times in this program, too — and slowly raise your arms. As you do, first bring them out to the side, then up. But stay aware of what your shoulders are doing, and stop whenever you feel them coming up, then bring your arms forward, away from your head. Readjust your shoulders down and wide, then continue raising your arms. Keep doing that until your hands are shoulder width apart. Unless you're very flexible, when your hands get to the top (don't bring them any closer than shoulder width apart) your arms will need to be forward of perpendicular [Fig.11]. Turn sideways to the mirror and compare your arm position to those below.

► **Tight**

MJ's arms come far forward, away from her head, almost 45 degrees off vertical [Fig.11]. Her shoulders are wide and her neck comfortable. And she doesn't need to arch her back to get her arms up as Susan did in Figure 9. If the point at which your arms are comfortably raised over your head is near this example and you can still widen your shoulder blades, your shoulders and chest are Tight.

► **Moderate**

Annie is able to take her arms overhead comfortably by taking them just forward of her head, about 30 degrees off vertical [Fig.12]. If your arms are close to hers, you have Moderate flexibility in your shoulders and chest. (Later on, you will notice that Annie's lower body is more flexible than her upper body.)

► **Flexible**

With her shoulders wide and her arms overhead, Susan's arms now form an almost vertical line [Fig.13]. If your posture looks like Susan's, your upper body is Flexible. Look at Figure 9 again. This is what happens if you try too hard to get your arms straight up and you aren't flexible enough: your back arches and your shoulders crunch. Don't force your arms straight overhead unless your body is truly flexible.

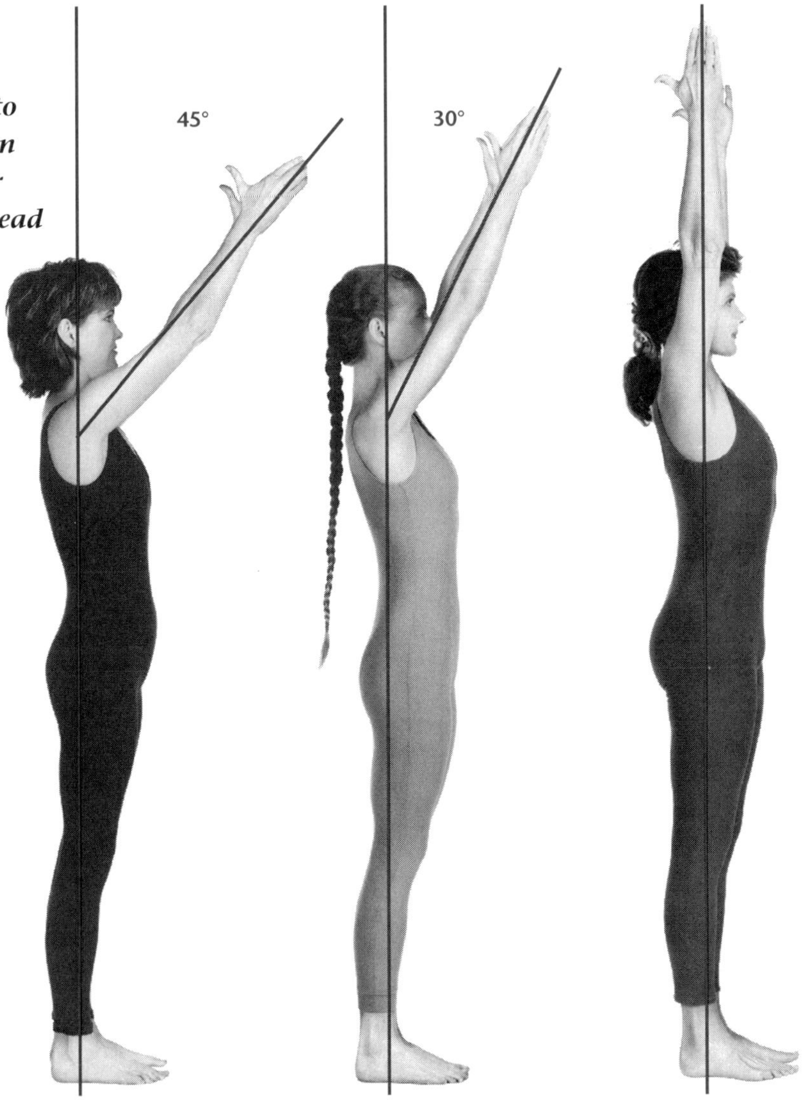

45°

30°

fig. 11

fig. 12

fig. 13

The Standing Hamstring Stretch Test

The Standing Hamstring Stretch tests the flexibility of the muscles, tendons, and ligaments in the rear of your body, particularly your hamstrings, as did the Lying Down Hamstring Stretch. It's also an indication of how flexible your hips and back are. The body type example you resemble here will also show you which example to use for the Forward Bend that follows in Part II and probably the Downward Facing Dog (also in Part II) as well.

CAUTION

This test duplicates a traditional Standing Forward Bend, a move that — as you're going to learn — is an inappropriate exercise for your body. This is only a test to determine your flexibility. I'll be teaching you the correct Forward Bend exercise in the Sun Salutation routine that follows in Part II.

While doing this test, don't force the stretch. Simply feel what is happening and then come up as directed.

Stand sideways to a mirror with your feet about two to three inches apart (wider if your knees touch). Now round your back and try to touch your toes (your shins if you're stiff or the floor next to the sides of your feet if you're very flexible). If your back hurts, take your hands higher up on your legs. If you're like most people, you'll feel some pain or significant tightness behind your knees (the tendons that attach your hamstring muscles to the back of your knees) and/or your calves and back of your ankles as you push further toward your toes. You may also feel a pull or strain in your lower back.

As you try it, don't hurt yourself, yet be fairly assertive in going down as far as you can but not pushing too much into pain. Then look in the mirror and see where you stopped.

How far are your shoulders from the floor? Your hands? Pay particular attention to where you feel the stretch. For most people, it will be behind the knees, calves, lower in the

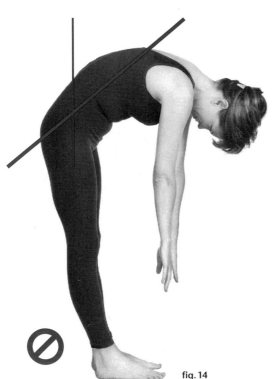

fig. 14

Achilles tendons, or worse yet, in the lower back. After you have done your Standing Hamstring Stretch, come back up, bending your knees just a little as you uncurl up, and relax for a moment and compare yourself with the following examples.

► *Tight*

In this example [Fig.14], MJ is reaching toward the floor but stops when she feels the pain behind her knees. Look at the line drawn through her sitting bones and the top of her hip bone; when you do a correct Forward Bend for your body type, this line should continue straight through your shoulders and head as well. Hers obviously doesn't, which shows that she's dropping down too far. If your Standing Hamstring Stretch looks like MJ's, a little higher or a little lower, consider your body type as Tight for the Forward Bend (that follows in Part II). This means that your hamstring and lower back muscles demonstrate limited elasticity (there is no judgment here; your body is just where it is). It's also an indication that you may be tight in other areas of your body.

Now look at Figures 15 and 16. MJ is touching her feet or ankles, but she's really pushing it and is feeling uncomfortable. Her back hurts and she feels pain behind her knees; in fact, there's pain running all the way up and down her legs. And look at that line running through her sitting bones and hips — it's still not coming close to lining up with her head and shoulders. Even though she might look flexible here, she's not.

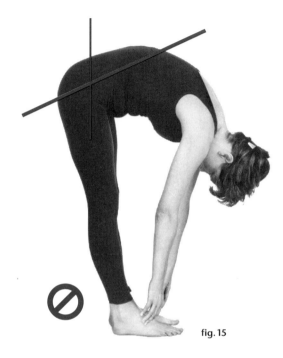

fig. 15

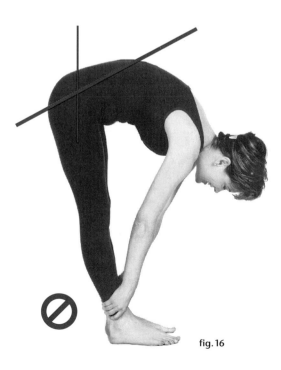

fig. 16

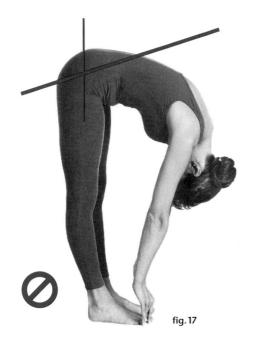

fig. 17

▶ Moderate

In this example, Susan [Fig.17] easily reaches her toes by rounding her back and dropping down. Again, although she looks very flexible, she's not — she feels pain behind her knees and in her back — but this is what a moderately flexible person looks like in the Standing Hamstring Stretch. The line drawn through her sitting bones and the top of the hip bone is closer to her head and shoulders; Susan has more pelvic rotation than MJ, and can come further down, still maintaining a straight spine. If your body comes close to this, your hamstrings and back are somewhat supple, and you can consider your general flexibility as Moderate.

▶ Flexible

In Figure 18, my hands are flat on the floor, my torso relaxes down and because of my flexibility, I am not feeling much of anything. If you get this far and you don't feel a hamstring stretch, lean forward a little on your feet; also lift your chest up and bring your ribs further down your legs. This should create a little more "action." In Figure 19, I am aggressively pulling into a traditional forward bend by pulling on my ankles. I feel more action (actually strain) behind my knees and in my lower back. In Figures 18 and 19, the line drawn through my sitting bones and hip bones (and my spine) still does not pass directly through my shoulders and head. If your Standing Hamstring Stretch looks like mine, the back side of your body is supple, and you will probably follow the Flexible example for most exercises.

In the above example, you should have felt at least some discomfort, or even some real pain, either behind the knees or in your lower back, or both. If you didn't, I would like you to go back now and push it just a little bit harder. But remember not to push it too hard or to make it hurt too much. Just experience a little discomfort.

You now have three indicators of how flexible your body is. Look at them and loosely average them together. If you were Tight in every test, you have a limited range of flexibility, and you need to approach this program patiently. If you push yourself, you may become frustrated or hurt. You'll want to start with the Tight example for all the exercises. Paradoxically, I've found that those students who type themselves Tight and nonaggressively approach the program ultimately understand and progress the quickest because they can feel the appropriate action much sooner than a flexible person. If you go slowly and allow your body to open up, within a few weeks you'll notice a considerable difference. Go back to the tests after a month of practice and see if your body has changed.

If you were Tight in the hamstring tests, and Moderate in the Arms Overhead test, you could go either way in the exercises, especially in those that combine elements of upper and lower body flexibility. I suggest always starting with the Tight example, then slowly move toward the Moderate examples when you're ready.

If you tested Flexible in all three, do not proceed with abandon. You need to learn the details of ExTension in order to tone your body, retain your flexibility, improve your strength and endurance, and avoid injuring and tightening soft tissue.

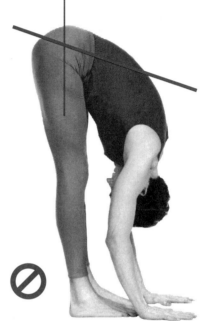

fig. 18

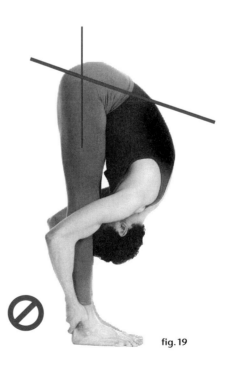

fig. 19

ASSESS YOUR PERSONALITY

The three personality types I've chosen to use are: Aggressive, Moderate, and Easygoing. You can probably type yourself by simply looking at the words, but be willing to take a hard, objective look beyond your initial reaction to them. I'm talking about internal aggression or passivity. You could be a very aggressive professional but laid back (even lazy) when it comes to helping yourself. Aggression is a survival mechanism and there's nothing wrong with it, except if it hurts you. In exercise, if you aggressively keep pushing past pain, ignoring what it could be doing to your body, it will ultimately slow you down and could even hurt you. And it's absolutely unnecessary. Let's look at these basic personality types.

Aggressive:

Always Pushing, Workaholic, an Obsessive Exerciser

Are you something of a control freak? Are you impatient and nervous? Do you get mad when something is clearly beyond your physical abilities? Did you feel frustrated if you couldn't do the more flexible tests? Did you keep pushing even though I told you not to? For the purposes of this book, consider yourself *Aggressive*. Some call it "Type A."

Moderate:

Balanced Between Work/Rest, a Moderate Exerciser

You may consider yourself somewhere in between, internally content but with a desire to improve. You are not lazy, but you respect and honor your limitations and will quit when appropriate. You have patience when moving toward your goals. I'd call you a *Moderate* personality.

Easygoing:

Laid Back, Passive, a Reluctant Exerciser

Are you resistant when it comes to working out or doing anything that takes a consistent physical effort? Do you take your time when moving toward goals? Did you buy this book reluctantly (or did someone give it to you as a gift and you're just now getting around to looking at it)? Do you talk a lot about not having the right motivation to exercise? When you do exercise, do you quit soon after starting? If so, you're what I call the *Easygoing* type.

Here's how to apply your personal profile to the exercises you're about to learn:

Aggressive Types

You need to back off. Pushing yourself through the pain you feel in these exercises will work against you. To allow tight or injured tissue to open up, you have to relax. If you push, you may cause or exacerbate pain, and pain will cause you to tense up. The muscles will not relax, and you're caught in a cycle of pain, causing contraction, causing further pain, causing further contraction (again, it's

Hilton's Law — learn more in Part III). Even if you think you can try harder, don't. Breathe deeply, relax, and trust that ExTension works. But you need to remind yourself constantly NOT to push.

You might ask yourself how you can progress and change if you simply accept where you are. Because that's how you will allow changes to happen — by intelligently allowing your body to open and then relax. I said, *intelligently*, not aggressively. This distinction is one of the hardest for aggressive individuals to grasp; but when you do, it will change your practice.

Naturally, you'll resist this whole concept. You think you'll become soft, lazy, lose your edge. But just the opposite will happen. You'll feel stronger and more energized than you ever have before. Read again the Foreword by fitness expert Molly Fox.

I have a student who's a very successful businesswoman. Extremely aggressive. When she first started learning ExTension, she was a slave to the form. She would do anything to make it look perfect. She kept remarking on how good her postures were becoming. Only one thing was wrong. She kept getting tighter and her back began hurting. Well, she pushed too hard and got hurt and had to back off and relearn the exercises. She had to readjust her approach to them; she needed to listen to what her body was telling her. After much discussion, she finally understood what I had been saying all along — that less, when done correctly, will get you more.

Since she readjusted her approach, her physical progress has been steady. But her personality change has been remarkable. All those around her have noticed a surge of vitality coupled with a new congeniality and a willingness to listen rather than to be continually directive. She has become more flexible both physically and emotionally. And she continues to be very competitive and successful. Experiment with it. Won't it be a relief to relax a little and still not give up your edge?

Moderate Types

If you're feeling energetic and ambitious, you can push your postures a bit. Strive to improve yourself. Just remember that pain is a message to avoid going any further. Some days you'll feel a little slower, a little tired, and you can simply back off, put in your time, and still receive significant benefits. You know — or you will know — when you're doing your best and when you're not. And it's not necessarily when you're "trying" the hardest.

Easygoing Types

You can practice ExTension lackadaisically and feel great. You will benefit and you don't have to sweat. You can just have fun with it, and that's fine. But if you want more out of ExTension, if you want to make some real changes in your body tone and in your energy level, you need to be assertive with these exercises. They may feel easy, so challenge yourself according to the directions. Push the edges. If the postures feel hard but not painful, hold on as long as you can and don't give up. But, if you hurt while doing them, you must back off. Next time, go right up to that point once more. Do a few extra repetitions. You'll be surprised how much you can get out of ExTension and how wonderful you'll feel because of it.

ARROWS INDICATE MOVEMENT

For some of the exercises that follow, you'll find explicit instructions for your personality type. For some exercises you'll simply see arrows indicating which direction you should be moving various parts of your body. If you're an aggressive type, you'll ease up on the direction of the arrows. If you tend to be more easygoing, follow the direction of the arrows, which will make these exercises more challenging. But as always, never push yourself to the point of pain.

Now you're ready to start exercising. Follow the instructions for your body type and keep the personality cues in mind, and this program will work. It's that simple. Do it and you'll get results.

PART II

THE EXTENSION PROGRAM

This program is different

from any other exercise program

you've ever done.

It may look like classes or books

that you've seen before.

But there's a big difference...

In the ExTension program, you will learn that you must first do less than you're used to doing or being told to do and that taking the time to let your body open up will get you more than by pushing yourself to try harder and harder.

By less, I mean less time, less effort, and less aggression. You can devote as few as 20 minutes a day to your body and achieve as much as or more than you would going to an hour-long class.

But more important, by practicing ExTension you'll learn that pushing yourself harder, trying to do things that are not yet within your capacity, *works against* you. Here's why.

When you strain in an exercise or yoga posture, you set up a chain reaction. Any time you feel pain in a joint or soft tissue — especially tendons and ligaments — you affect the surrounding muscles and skin. And you can extend this principle to apply to the fascia, which wraps throughout your inner body — your organs and glands — and is intertwined throughout and over each muscle. As I explained in "The ExTension Principles," I believe that once you irritate fascia, it tightens up. It holds all the injury your body has ever experienced. As you grow older, fascia gets even tighter, tightening muscle, inhibiting internal movement, making you feel tired and sluggish. You feel a nonspecific fatigue, even pain, that sometimes makes it impossible to relax and uncomfortable to exercise.

The goal of this program is gently, progressively, to release the tension in your overall fascia, soft tissue, and joints by isolating each exercise in specific areas of your body. You learn yoga-based exercises, called "postures" and "poses," that address particular areas of your body. They're designed to allow to you to breathe very deeply and fully, which enhances the exercise and makes you feel fabulous. Without pain and without strained effort, your physiology opens up and your flexibility is increased.

The specific muscle group that you're going to read about the most is your hamstrings, those muscles in the back part of your upper thigh. Most of the exercises in ExTension stretch those hamstrings, and again and again you'll be instructed to isolate the stretch to the belly, or thickest part, of that muscle group. Learning to stretch there correctly will help your hamstrings to loosen up, which in turn eases low back pain and may ease chronic pain in other parts of your body, too.

A secondary but equally important goal is to help you let go of trying to look like a particular ideal while you exercise. Whether you're trying to mimic a teacher or an example in a book, you're doing someone else's exercise and could be setting yourself up for frustration, injury, and defeat. In this book you'll learn how to do each exercise based on your own physiology, which you will have already assessed.

And no matter how tight or flexible you are, you will find yourself represented in the photographs that illustrate each pose.

I believe that *trying* — trying to look like someone else, trying to accomplish a physical task that is beyond your limits — is responsible for discouragement, pain, and even injury in exercise classes. Let's say, for example, that you're a 40-year-old woman in a regular aerobics class. Your instructor, a 25-year-old nymph, tells you to "try to touch your toes" and demonstrates. You follow, rounding your back over and reaching for your toes. You find that you can only reach your shins. You look around, start feeling embarrassed, and try harder. It hurts, and you still can't reach your toes. You feel discouraged and resolve to try harder next time. If there is a next time.

That's why I strive never to use the word "try."

Before You Start

As I said before, the best way to use this book is to read it all the way through first. It's important for you to understand why you may be approaching exercise reluctantly or regularly injuring yourself and why this program is different and will work better for you.

Then familiarize yourself with each separate exercise, the first of which is simple deep breathing, followed by learning how to stand on your own two feet. The book will teach you the individual poses for a sequence called Sun Salutations, separately at first, then you will learn how to put them together in a beautiful combination that will become the foundation for your physical and emotional well-being. You can practice them slowly or you can eventually challenge (without aggressively pushing) yourself for even more physical benefits. The rest of the exercises, Standing Postures, Floor Exercises, and Relaxation will follow and complete your daily workout. And once you understand the system, all this can be done in as little as 20 minutes a day.

For each exercise, read the general directions and cautions thoroughly. Experiment with the preparatory instructions and read about what you may expect to feel. Then find the illustration for your physical type (Tight, Moderate, or Flexible) and test out the exercise. Keep in mind that the physical types are just guidelines and you may fall somewhere in between. You may also find that for one exercise you will feel more comfortable following the specifications for a Tight body while for another your form might look more like a Flexible profile.

After you've gotten your general positioning down, check out the Fine-Tuning boxes for extra details on the exercise and to reinforce your good form. These are the details that will add depth to this program. The more you learn, the more you will be open to learn. It's sort of like a math class. Once you get level one, you can go on to level two — and once you get your basic form down, the finer details will open up the deeper levels and your knowledge will expand.

And don't forget your Attitude Adjustment details. Usually, you can simply look at the arrows you see on the illustrations, and use them to adjust the exercise according to your personality. For some of the exercises, you will find detailed adjustments in addition to the more general "arrow" adjustments.

Go through the physical practice, then finish with a session of relaxation. Even if it's just for a few moments, it's important to lie down, contain the energy and rejuvenation you've generated, and then go on with the rest of your day.

What You'll Need

The Sun Salutations and the standing exercises are best done on a hardwood floor because you can use the lines of the boards to align your hands and feet. If you have a tile or other hard surface, you might want to stand on a carpet remnant, cut slightly longer than your height and about two to three feet wide. Or you can work on a thin, non-slip mat called a sticky mat. It does just what it says: It sticks to the floor and creates a slight friction that keeps your hands and feet from sliding. If your floors are slippery, you'll need it for the standing postures. These mats may be ordered from various vendors advertising in *Yoga Journal*, a monthly magazine (see Resources in Appendix VI).

For floor exercises, a firm carpet is fine, as long as it's not deep, soft pile or shag. Thick or soft exercise mats are not desirable, because you sink into them too much, and your spine will not be able to lengthen and lift.

Some of the lying-down work requires that you totally relax your neck and shoulders. If this is difficult when you're flat on your back (you'll learn how to determine this later, in the Three-Part Breath), you'll need either a large folded towel or a piece of carpet sample that can be folded between one and three inches thick.

If you tend to be tight in the exercises, you'll also need a small footstool, bench, chair or stack of books for lying-down exercises and Downward Facing Dog (page 92). For the Side Twist (page 156), keep two firm pillows or two small stacks of folded bath towels nearby.

Wear comfortable clothing. When you're starting out, it helps to wear shorts or tights so that you can see what your legs and knees are doing. Always work barefoot. You might be tempted always to use a mirror in your practice. I encourage you to use a mirror initially in order to check out your alignment. But if you always use a mirror, it will focus your attention away from what you are feeling to what you are seeing. And only when you *feel* what is happening in your own body will you be able to progress appropriately.

Are you ready? Let's begin.

THE THREE-PART BREATH

In this program, you want to strive for deep, unrestricted breathing during every exercise. Deep breathing is crucial. Anything that restricts your breathing works against you. This is another good reason for wearing loose clothing while practicing this program. As you will soon learn, doing many of the exercises wrong will restrict your breathing.

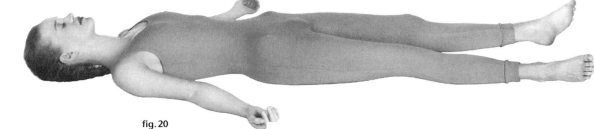

fig. 20

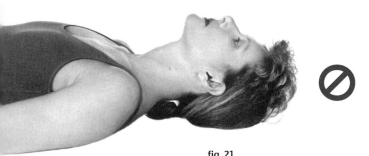

fig. 21

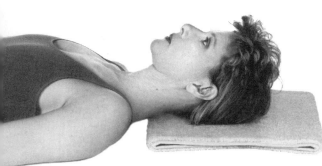

fig. 22

Many stress-management experts teach diaphragmatic breathing, which focuses on the diaphragm, your major respiratory muscle, to deepen and lengthen the breath. Here, for several reasons, you're going to learn the three-part breath, which also involves your middle and upper chest:

1. It deepens your breathing, which helps you to hold the exercises longer.
2. There's a direct connection between the nervous system and the breath — a deep breath soothes and relaxes you — so your body will relax and respond quicker.
3. It increases your endurance.
4. Smaller respiratory muscles, such as the intercostals (tiny muscles between the ribs) and other minor muscles of respiration, are often neglected. Three-part breathing expands and conditions them, allowing your breath to flow more easily.
5. Some of the postures you will learn in more advanced programs contract your diaphragm, making it hard to expand. The three-part breath teaches you to breathe into other areas of your chest and back.

Lie down on your back with your head on the floor [Fig. 20]. We're aiming for complete relaxation here, so notice if you experience any tightness in your neck, shoulders, or chest.

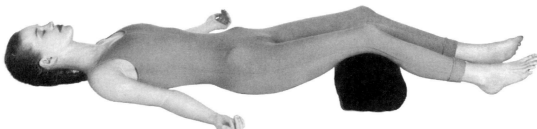

fig. 23

Actually, most beginners to ExTension don't (this is because of a nifty little mechanism called "habituation" which will be discussed later on). Does your chin come higher than your eyes [Fig.21]? You can check this out by having a friend look at the relationship between your chin and your eyes when you lie flat with your head on the floor. If so, place a firmly folded towel, blanket, or, my personal favorite, a folded carpet sample (nothing higher than one and a half to two inches) under your head [Fig.22]. If you don't use some support, it will be impossible for you to relax; your entire body (especially your upper body) will remain tense. Test it out; does it feel better? If not, use a lower support or just don't use one.

At first, it may be uncomfortable to lie with your legs out long. If it is, keep your knees bent, feet flat on the floor. Or, better yet, place a pillow or rolled carpet sample under your knees [Fig.23] or rest your legs and feet on a chair [Fig.24]. After a few weeks of practice you may be able to lie flat on the floor without needing to use head or leg supports, but use them whenever it feels better with than without them.

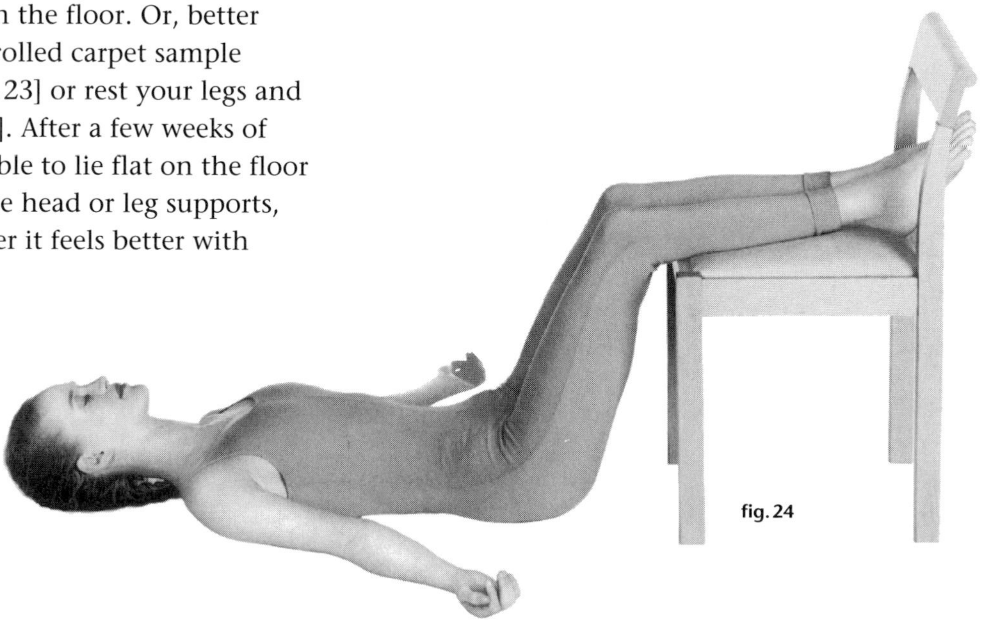

fig. 24

Now, put both hands flat on your belly, fingertips touching [Fig.25]. Inhale deeply but softly through your nose, if possible, and feel your abdominal area fill your hands. As you exhale — also through your nose, if possible, allow your belly to drop downward toward the floor. Breathing through your nose evokes a beneficial response from your nervous system. If it's difficult or uncomfortable, just breathe through your mouth for now. Soon you'll be able to breathe through your nose more comfortably. Make the exhalation last longer than the inhalation, but don't force your breath out. Rather, allow it to feel soft and comfortable, not strained. Do this until your breath flows smoothly and easily, without jerkiness.

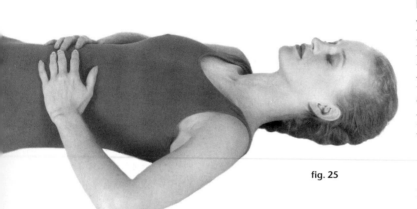

fig. 25

Move your hands up to your rib cage [Fig.26]. Cup your ribs with your hands, fingertips touching again. Breathe in deeply, so your fingertips begin to move apart as you inhale and move back together again as you exhale. If you do not feel as if your fingertips are moving now, you will later as your intercostal muscles become more flexible. Inhale, then exhale again, allowing the exhalation to last about twice as long as the inhalation, keeping it gentle and easy, moving your fingers together again. Do this until it feels smooth and comfortable.

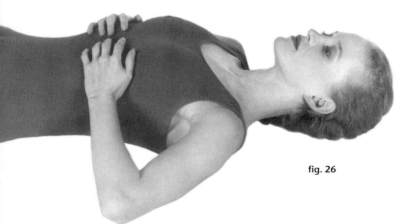

fig. 26

Finally, move your hands above your breast line to your upper chest [Fig.27]. Keep your belly still and breathe only into your hands on your upper chest. Some people initially find it difficult to feel any movement; just do the best you can, but of course, don't strain. Inhale, observe if your hands move up during inhalation, and then exhale, observing if they move downward again.

Once you can practice the three parts of this breath easily, put them together within the same breath. Start with your hands low on your belly. Inhale, and as you fill each section, move your hands up to the next. Abdomen, middle ribs, upper chest. Exhale and reverse the process, feeling each section empty as you move your hands down. Upper chest, middle ribs, abdomen. Repeat this sequence a few times with exhalation lasting longer than inhalation.

With practice you'll become adept at controlling your breath whether lying down, sitting, or standing. And you won't need to use your hands.

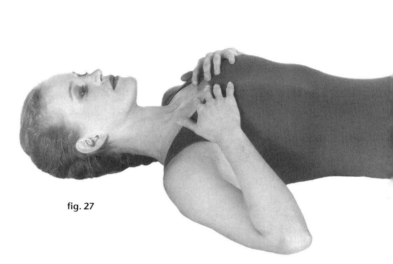

fig. 27

Do this three-part breathing often, any time during the day. Sitting at your desk as stress piles up. Waiting in line. At home after a tiring day. In bed before going to sleep. You will be amazed at how quickly it will de-stress and relax you. It works as well as or better than a glass of wine or beer, and without any side effects.

Remember that holding your breath holds in tension; whether you're at work, exercising, or resting. I'll be reminding you of that often.

One more thing. As you "relearn" how to breathe and develop a deeper sense of your breath flowing evenly and deeply without effort, you will experience a deeper appreciation for life and what this program will bring you. Breathing beats the alternative. Breathing deeply can make you happier.

STANDING

Standing is something most people take for granted. But in ExTension as well as in everyday life, you really can't afford to. In fact, the way you stand may be responsible for the fatigue you feel every day.

Find a full-length mirror, and stand sideways to it. Look at your posture. Now imagine a fishing line, with a sinker on the end of it, passing through the center of your ear all the way to the ground. If your body were perfectly in balance and aligned, what we call "in plumb," that line would drop right down the centerline of your body: the center of your neck, shoulder, hip, knee, and ankle (just like the "plumb line" in Bachin's "Skeletal System" on page 189). Does your head come forward of the plumb line? Your pelvis? Your knees?

Being out of plumb just a little means that your skeletal system is no longer supporting your body upright, but that muscles in the front of you — or the back of you — have to work harder just to keep you from falling over. If one part of you is out of balance and "off the plumb," another part of you must take over to compensate.

You can test this by exaggerating some common misalignments. First, lock your knees and lean your body way forward [Fig.28]. If you hold this position and exaggerate your head coming just a little farther forward, you'll sense the muscles in the front of your body becoming tight, including your shins and ankles. Now slouch and thrust the top of your pelvis forward [Fig. 29]. As you throw weight back on your heels, feel how that loads up your back. And just plain slouching [Fig.30] can load up all of these areas.

If you chronically stand any of these ways, just a little bit, your body has moved off the plumb. And without even knowing it, your muscles are constantly tightening and fighting simply to help you stay erect. After just one day of this constant compensation, you will feel fatigued. After years you will get used to it, but you will feel tired all the time. Your body has become *habituated* to the discomfort.

But when you practice ExTension regularly, the muscles of the back of your body move into balance with the muscles in the front of your body and you can move closer and closer to the plumb [Fig.31].

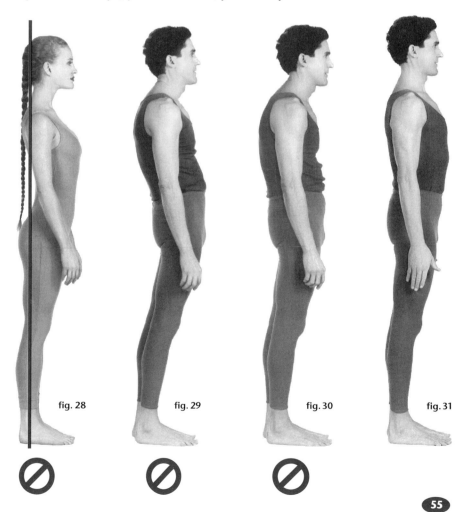

fig. 28   fig. 29   fig. 30   fig. 31

The Mountain Pose: A New Way of Standing

This chapter shows you how to stand correctly on your own two feet. Your feet and legs will form the foundation of your posture, which, like the foundation of a tall building, will allow you to withstand the stresses that confront you.

FINE-TUNING

Many people have flat feet or dropped arches, [Fig. 33] which causes the knees to rotate inward and can weaken the standing exercises which follow. If you're one of these people, you can learn to "activate" your feet, which will make all the standing exercises become more powerful (after several years of using this method, I have corrected my flat feet). Even if you don't have dropped arches, activating your feet still dramatically affects your legs and spine in the standing poses.

Here's how: While standing, stay in contact with the floor on all four of those points and consciously lift your arch/instep up [Fig. 34]. To help learn how to lift your arches, lift your toes off the floor while keeping the inner balls and inner heels of your feet pressing down; then lift your arches up. Feel as if there is a marble directly under your arch and you want lift your arch up and away from that marble. Lifting your arches helps your knees to stay parallel.

Stand with your feet almost parallel, two to three inches apart, the toes just a bit wider than your heels. As you stand, there are four points on each foot on which you want to feel weight; the inner heel, the outer heel, the inner ball mount, and the outer ball mount [Fig. 32]. Just as four tires on a car hold the road, you should stand so that you feel equal weight on each foot and on each of those four points. It's important to practice on a hard surface — a firm carpet or hardwood floor — because you need to be able to feel the

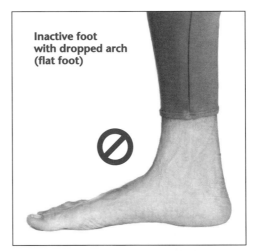

Inactive foot with dropped arch (flat foot)

fig. 33

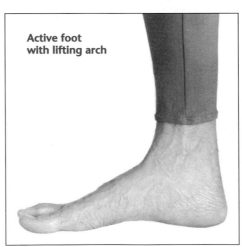

Active foot with lifting arch

fig. 34

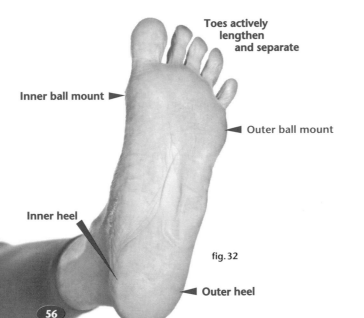

Toes actively lengthen and separate

Inner ball mount ►

◄ Outer ball mount

Inner heel

fig. 32

◄ Outer heel

balanced weight on your feet so that the rest of your body, especially your spine, can extend. Remember, *ExTension releases tension.*

Standing up straight in the Mountain pose is important, but it doesn't mean throwing your shoulders back, arching your back, or sticking out your buttocks. Instead, imagine that someone has his hand over your head [Fig.35]. By lengthening your spine, bringing your ears away from your shoulders and gently lifting with your rib cage, feel yourself growing taller and rising into the palm of that imaginary hand.

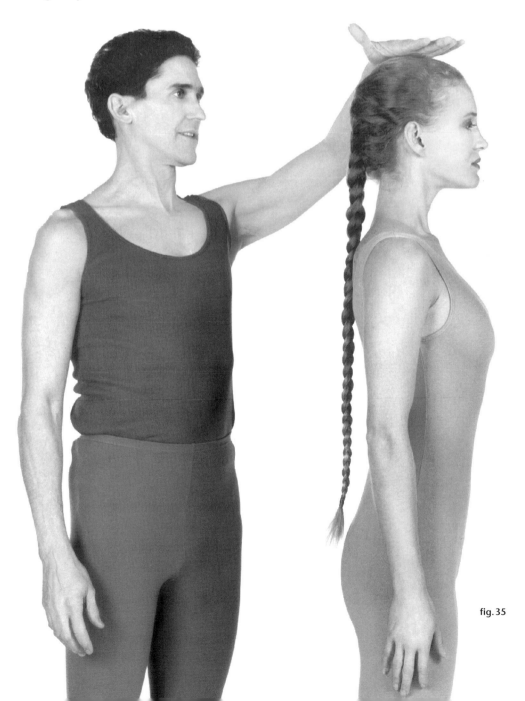

fig. 35

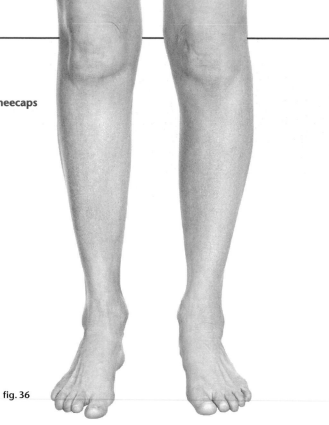

"Lifted" Kneecaps

fig. 36

FINE-TUNING

Perhaps you have a hard time keeping your feet near parallel — it feels better with them turned out — that's because your deep inner hip rotator muscles are tight. You'll soon be learning an exercise called Gluteal Rolling, which will help release this tightness and restore balance to these deep hip muscles. But for now, just let your feet turn out as far as they feel comfortable, always keeping the intention of rotating them toward parallel.

Also, some people (especially women) try to minimize their behinds by "tucking in" their buttocks. By doing that (and you've probably been told to do so in dance and exercise classes), you squeeze out your natural lower back, or lumbar curve. Don't do it; a lumbar curve is crucial to good, comfortable posture and a healthy back.

Never lock or push your knees back — you can irritate knee tendons and ligaments. Instead, always lift the kneecaps; do not allow them to sag [Fig. 36, lifted kneecaps, Fig. 37, dropped kneecaps]. Lifting your kneecaps is a subtle move, but if you keep practicing, it will get easier and more comfortable.

Before continuing, let's experiment with one more thing. Standing tall and relaxed, take some deep breaths. As you inhale deeply, but gently, notice the volume of air you can take

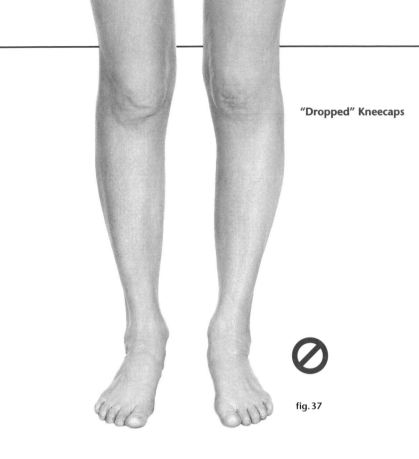

"Dropped" Kneecaps

fig. 37

CAUTION

If you have a history of knee problems, you may find it difficult to keep your feet near parallel. If your knees hurt, turn your feet out a little to release the discomfort. You might need to keep your knees slightly bent as well. After you've been practicing for a while, and your leg muscles become more balanced, it will be easier to keep your feet parallel.

into your lungs. Now, slump way down as if you were very tired or depressed and take another deep inhalation. Can you feel the difference in your lung capacity? Come back up. Standing tall now, pretend that you feel happy and light on your feet. Take another inhalation. Feels deeper, doesn't it? Even more important, though, is that a deeper breath flushes out carbon dioxide and lactic acid and brings in oxygen which is crucial in helping your muscles recover from the effects of exercise.

Mountain pose is the foundation and starting place for most of the exercises that follow. Although good posture makes you look and feel younger, it is important to remember that you can't force yourself into it. You'll find that as you practice ExTension, your body becomes more balanced and it becomes easier to "stay on the plumb." Just keep at it and it will happen.

SUN SALUTATIONS

THE FOUNDATION OF EXTENSION

Thousands of years ago, the ancients devised a sequence of movements to wake up their bodies and give thanks for the rising of the sun each day. The result: the Sun Salutation, a form of exercise that works every major muscle group of the body. The classical routine is familiar to anyone who has done yoga before. The ancient Eastern practitioners, however, had none of the tensions of our modern Western culture. They were extremely flexible and had no problem with the deep bending and extending movements of the spine and joints.

Our Western bodies are not so fortunate. The ancients were strict vegetarians and spent the majority of their lives in humble surroundings without the benefit of today's conveniences such as frozen, prepackaged, processed and fast foods, coffee and ice cream, automobiles and air travel, regular office hours, and television and soft furniture. Yet the classical Sun Salutation has been taught basically unchanged for centuries.

ExTension simplifies and demystifies these exercises to be easier on our Western bodies. The Sun Salutation practiced the ExTension way is a wonderful routine that tones, stretches, and flexes your whole body, without pain or strain. And it's extremely adaptable. You can do the movements slowly and quietly to promote a deep sense of relaxation — a "meditation in action." Done in repetition, they become a complete workout that will condition your cardiovascular system as well as your muscles. As the routine becomes more familiar you can even build up a powerful sweat.

Sun Salutations can also be used to warm up your body for regular workouts, whatever your discipline or sport, or as a cool-down after a workout to keep your body from knotting up. I do a few every morning as a warm-up for my daily advanced yoga practice. Then, about two to three times a week, I go through 20 to 25 minutes of quick Sun Salutation repetitions for cardiovascular fitness.

Each separate exercise, or "pose," within the Sun Salutation routine is fully explained so that you can really learn and master it. You then can put them together for the flowing Sun Salutation sequence. Or you may decide to practice each pose separately, isolating and holding the stretches and flexes for as long as you like. Either way, you need to understand each movement fully before practicing it, especially if you're going to use them in brisk repetition for cardiovascular enhancement. First, go slowly and master the individual poses within the routine.

FINE-TUNING

A note before you start: Since you've already typed yourself as Tight, Moderate, or Flexible, you may be tempted to follow only the example for your body type. Don't. You'll notice that different models will be used to illustrate various examples.

Sometimes I will be demonstrating the Tight adaptation and sometimes I will be the Flexible or Moderate example. In the Sun Salutation sequence, Annie is used as the Moderate example, but she actually shows more hip flexibility than I do when I demonstrate the Flexible sequence. This is quite common, and it's why you need to start with your body type's representation, then adapt it to how you're feeling. Back off, or challenge yourself. And take a minute before each exercise either to visualize or to think about what you're going to do; then do it.

The Arm Flap

The first exercise is called the Arm Flap. It looks like simply raising your arms up over your head. Seems like an easy enough thing to do, but as you learned in the Arms Overhead Test in Part I, if you do it without thinking, and without some adjustment for your flexibility, you could seriously crunch your shoulders and tighten your neck and set up a cycle of tension and pain.

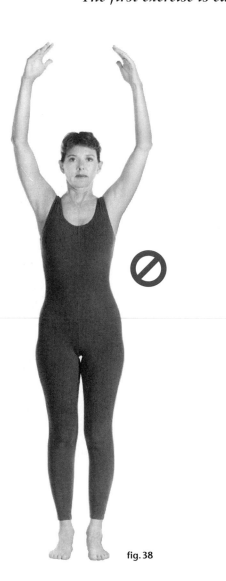

fig. 38

Preparation and Proofs: A Little Anatomy

Stand in front of your mirror and raise your arms up over your head a couple of times, without any of the hand or shoulder details you learned in the tests in Part I. Meaning: Keep your arms and hands relaxed and deactivated this time, as Susan demonstrates in Figure 38. Inhale as you bring your soft hands and arms out and up; exhale as your lower them. Notice what happens to your shoulders. If you're like most people, they will be lifting and crunching into the base of your neck and upper back. Maybe just a little, maybe a lot, but lifting and crunching just the same. It may hurt or it may feel tight; but remember, any degree of tightness or pain in your neck tells you that there's something wrong with the way you're moving and there is a way to do it differently.

Now for some additional details: With your hands down at your sides, just shrug your shoulders up toward your ears [Fig. 39]. Really scrunch them and take note of how it feels. Your neck probably feels tense, your shoulders tight, and perhaps even your breathing feels a little restricted.

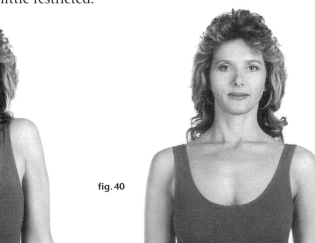

fig. 39   fig. 40

The ExTension Arm Flap

As you learned in Part I, if you feel (or see) your shoulders hunching up when you extend your arms overhead, you must take your arms forward — as much as you need to — as they come overhead. (Check out the position for your body type, pages 64–65.)

Now do the Arm Flap: inhale, stretch your arms out to the side (keep your hands active — see "Fine-Tuning" detail on page 65 — and palms up) and then up over your head. Adjust, move, then adjust again, so that you can keep your shoulders down and your shoulder blades wide and feel no tightness in your neck or upper back. When your arms are up over your head [Fig.41], your neck and shoulders should feel as comfortable as they do when your arms are down [Fig.40].

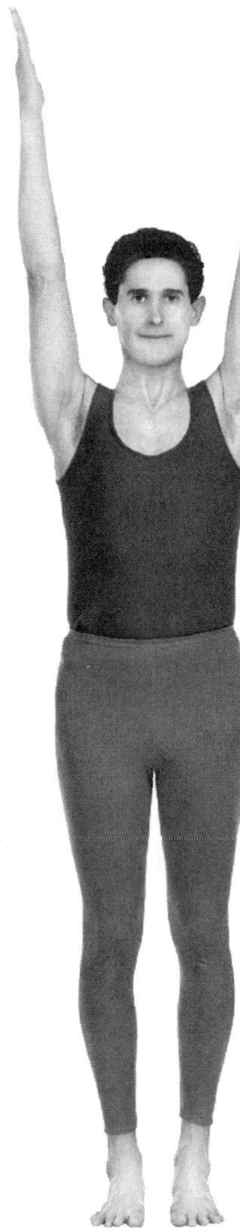

End with your palms facing each other no closer than shoulder width apart and keep your shoulders down. Conjure up an image of DaVinci's body within a circle [Fig.42]. Then exhale and lower your arms, moving them out and away from your body, keeping your hands active. You'll end up with your palms down.

Do this about three to six times. Really extend your arms up over your head, keeping your hands active all the way up and all the way down (remember to keep your shoulders down and wide). Inhale while you take the arms up, and exhale while you take the arms down. Rest a few moments and observe how you feel. Then take your arms up and down again, but this time, keep them soft as Susan does in Figure 38, paying no attention to your breathing.

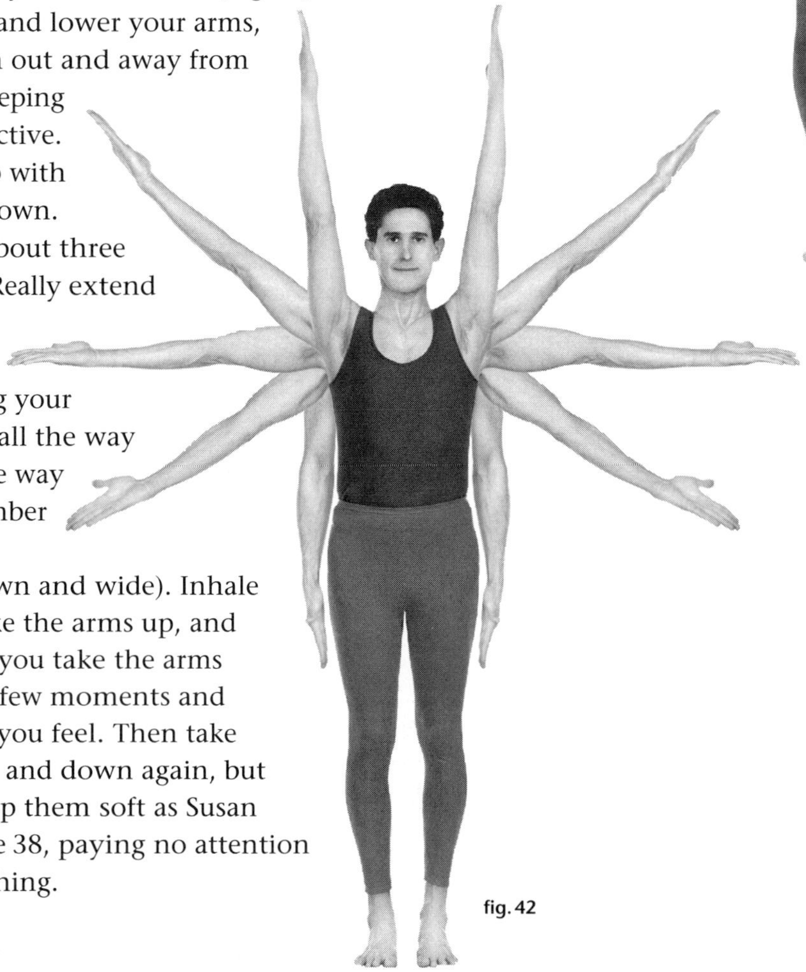

fig. 41

fig. 42

CAUTION

Remember: Don't hold your breath during any of the ExTension exercises. Holding your breath inhibits the physical benefits and the mental relaxation that is available to you. Learn to slow down your inhalations and exhalations, which, when coordinated with your Arm Flaps, will slow down their movements as well.

Notice how much better the movement feels when you stretch your arms out from your center and breathe correctly. Activating your hands and arms is similar to activating your feet and legs as you learned in Principle #5: *ExTension Releases Tension.* While doing the program, activate your feet and legs whenever you are standing by pulling up on your kneecaps, feeling all four points on your feet pressing down and lifting the arches of your feet.

Check below for the example of the Arm Flap for your body type.

▶ *Tight*

As you rotate your arms up, keep them far forward of your head (about 30 to 45 degrees off vertical), to keep shoulders from hunching up [Fig. 43]. Really extend your arms out from center before raising them overhead. Deep inhalation up and deep exhalation down.

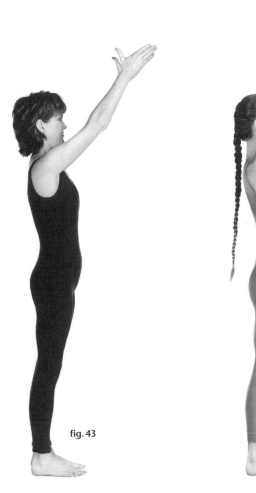

fig. 43

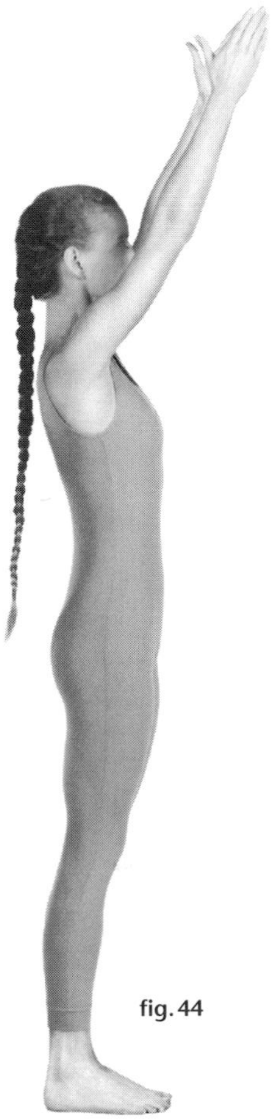

fig. 44

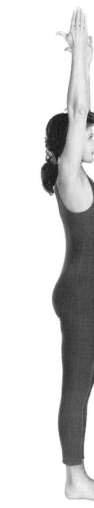

fig. 45

► *Moderate*

Arms rotate up slightly forward of head (about 20 to 30 degrees off vertical), enough to keep shoulders from tightening up [Fig. 44]. Active hands, extended arms. Deep, soft, slow inhalation up and exhalation down coordinating movement of arms with breath.

► *Flexible*

Arms rotate vertical (directly over your head) [Fig. 45]. Keep your hands and arms active throughout the Arm Flap and be sure to coordinate long, deep, smooth inhalations and exhalations with the movement of your arms. When your arms are up over your head, double check yourself by looking in a mirror to see if you're forcing the movement by lifting your shoulders or arching your back. You may think of yourself as flexible, and it may be hard to admit that you can't bring your arms up to vertical while adhering to the details. Remember, adapting this or any exercise doesn't make it any less effective.

FINE-TUNING

"Hands Active" mode [Figs. 46 and 47]: With your fingers together, stretch your thumb away from the rest of your hand so that it's perpendicular to your other fingers. Don't hyperextend your hand so much that the fingers start to bend back, but keep all the fingers extended and in line with your wrists. The active hand helps increase the extension in your arms and torso, increases the effectiveness of the exercise, and decreases tension and fatigue.

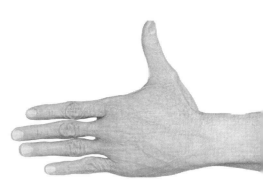

fig. 46

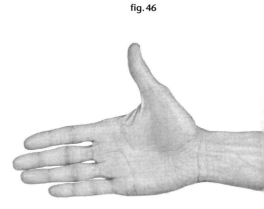

fig. 47

WHAT YOU'LL FEEL

The extension you're creating in your hands and arms will make this movement feel very graceful and flowing with no tightness in your neck, shoulders, or upper back. Feel or visualize yourself grounding your feet firmly into the floor and stretching as tall as you can, lifting your ribs up (but not forward) from your hips. Create a balance between the muscles in the front and back of your body, feeling your arms, legs, and spine extend equally.

The Forward Bend

The usual way of doing a standing forward bend is simply to round your back, bend over with your legs straight, and try to touch your toes. You tested it in the introduction to help you determine your flexibility. Do it again now, and notice what you feel. Go down just until you feel a pull in your legs, your back, or both. Keep your legs straight. If you're really flexible, you may have to grab your ankles and pull your head toward your feet [Fig.48].

Pay particular attention to where you feel the stretch in your legs and in your back. For most people, it will be behind the knees or in the Achilles tendon in the calves. And quite a few people feel it in their lower backs. Come back up now, bending your knees as you round up, relax, and read on.

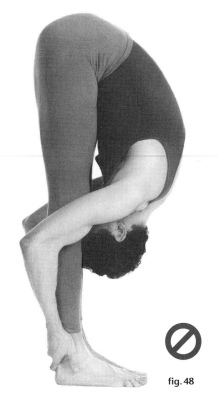

fig. 48

Preparation and Proofs: A Little Anatomy

Let me explain what's wrong with the usual Forward Bend. Bend your right arm and "make a muscle." Now grab the thickest part of that muscle, your biceps, with your left hand [Fig.49]. Feel how fleshy that area — the belly of a muscle — is? That's because it's full of blood, which means it's very resilient and able to recover quickly if injured or overstretched. Next, move your hand closer to the elbow and notice how the belly of the muscle changes, tapers down, and becomes small and hard [Fig.50]. The muscle is merging into tendon, which in turn attaches to bone. All of your muscles, including the hamstrings, do the

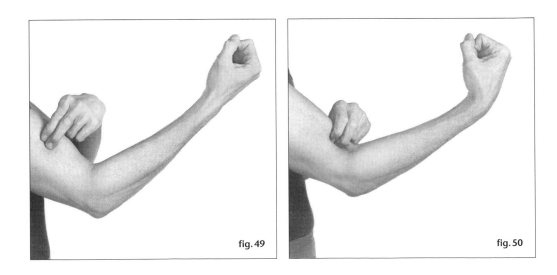

fig. 49   fig. 50

same thing. If you isolate a stretch in the belly of a muscle, you will enhance your flexibility without hurting yourself. But if you take the stretch into tendons, you may cause irritation which can lead to tendonitis. If you're young and healthy, a tendonitis might heal within three to six weeks; as you get older, however, it usually takes longer. If you stretch deeply into your joints, you could overstretch ligaments; if a ligament is injured, surgery is usually your only recourse.

Turn again to Bachin's "Muscular System" on page 188. Look at the lower back. It looks just like tendon tissue, not muscle tissue — dense, light-colored, with not much blood circulation, and therefore similarly tough to heal if injured or overstressed.

To summarize, *when you keep your legs locked straight and round your back trying to touch the floor, you're actually stretching tendon and the denser tissues of the lower back instead of hamstring muscle.* Since the areas of the low back and knee tendons are so difficult to heal when injured, the goal of ExTension is to stretch your body appropriately by isolating, at least initially, the action of each exercise in muscle, not tendon or low back tissue. You also want to *avoid* bouncing as you stretch (called ballistic stretching), which often leads to muscle, tendon, or ligament injuries.

I want to show you two more things about the traditional standing Forward Bend. Raise your arms up overhead, then bend forward from your waist with a flat back [Fig. 51]. As you fold over, can you feel a strain in your lower back? That's because as your arms move overhead, the "load" to your lower back increases by at least four times than when your hands stay on your hips. Look at the arrow in Figure 51 (page 67). That's where the entire

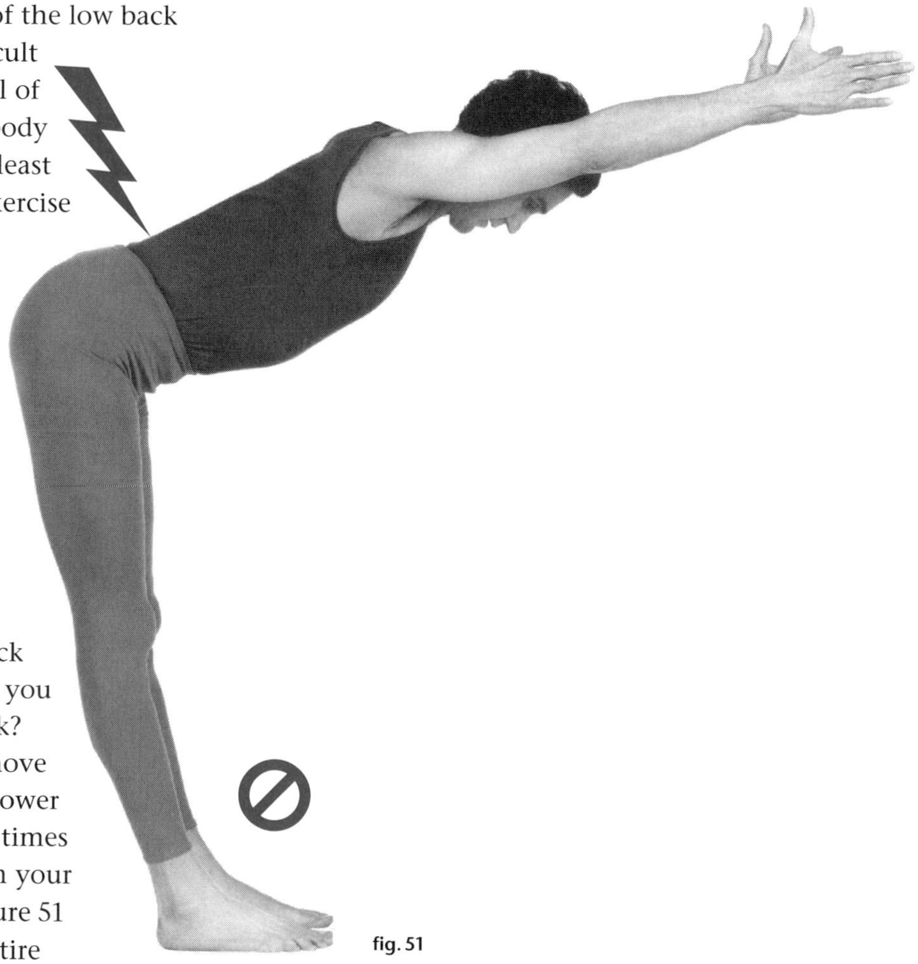

fig. 51

load from this exercise is taken. If you have a weak back, a current injury, or predisposition to injury, a chain reaction of pain-contraction-pain sets in. There is no way to correct this — just don't do it.

Come down into a traditional rounded-back Forward Bend one last time. Earlier, you learned that when you stand up straight, you can breathe more deeply than when you stand with a slump. You also learned in the ExTension Principles how important a deep breath is. In other words, you learned that exercises which inhibit your breath cannot be nearly as good for you as exercises that enhance your breath.

So, for the last time, go on now into the standing Forward Bend with a rounded back. Push down as low as you can. Not only will you experience discomfort behind your legs and perhaps in your lower back, but notice how your breath becomes inhibited. Then, bend your knees slightly and slowly stand up.

The ExTension Forward Bend

Let's now explore how *less gets you more* (remember Principle #3?) by learning a better way of bending forward. This time, we are going to isolate the stretch (action) right in the center of your hamstrings.

First, stand in Mountain pose, with your feet nearly parallel about two to three inches apart, weight balanced equally on both feet (forward and rear, left and right). Place your hands on your hips and extend your spine long. Center and relax your head on your neck by turning it side to side a few times. Now, keeping your knees *slightly* bent, slowly bend forward from your hips.

Lift up on your sitting bones and tailbone (imagine you have duck feathers that you want to show off). Only go down as far as you need to in order to feel the action (a stretch) in the center of your hamstring muscles, not the tendons behind your knees. If you feel discomfort behind your knees or in your back, take your torso up higher, and then, if you still feel discomfort behind your knees, bend them a little more. You may only need to rotate slightly forward before you feel a hamstring stretch; if so, you don't need to go down any lower.

Breathing deeply, lengthen your spine even further by feeling as if your belly is growing longer, your lower back naturally arching more (you must be careful here because overarching your back will cause pain). Your shoulders should move higher from the floor when your spine grows longer. This movement should increase the stretch of your hamstrings.

Notice a few things while you hold this posture as compared to before when you rounded your back down and dropped your hands toward the floor. Now you can isolate the stretch in the center of your hamstrings. Now you can breathe much more deeply. Now you don't feel that discomfort or pain behind your knees or in your back. And now you are actually doing *less* movement because you are much farther from the floor. Less, when done correctly, will always bring you more — less pain and discomfort and more accurate stretching. You're going to prove this over and over as you learn these exercises.

When you're ready to come out of this standing Forward Bend, don't just lift your shoulders to straighten up; this crunches your spine. Rather, think about initiating the rotation from your hips and pelvis, not from your shoulders. Move your whole torso as a single unit, keeping the integrity of your long spine and natural lumbar curve. Keep your knees slightly bent, your hands on your hips, and inhale on the way up to your standing position (Mountain pose). Then exhale, relax, and quietly deep breathe.

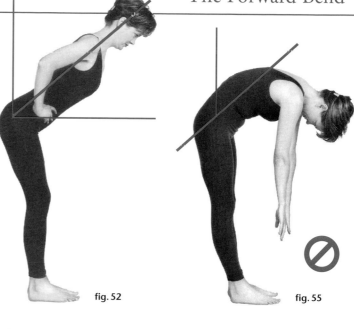

fig. 52

fig. 55

Here's how your forward bend will look, depending on your physical profile. Compare the lines drawn through the sitting bones, hips, shoulders, and head here [Figs. 52, 53, 54] with the lines in Figures 55, 56, and 57. Although the angles of the lines are about the same, Figures 52, 53, and 54 show the forward bend that is correct for each body type; notice how in each illustration, the spine is straight (not rounded); the hips, sitting bones, shoulders, and head are aligned; in Figures 55, 56, and 57, they are not.

▶ **Tight**

Body is about 45 degrees from vertical [Fig. 52]. Back is long, head neutral. Hands on hips, knees are bent just enough to feel the action or stretch in your hamstrings, not the tendons behind your knees. Hold for about two to four long, slow, complete inhalations and long, deep exhalations. Come up rotating from the pelvis, and repeat if you like. If you do not clearly feel an isolated hamstring stretch, note the Caution, below.

▶ **Moderate**

Body is about 60 degrees from vertical (not quite horizontal with the floor) [Fig. 53]. Back is long, tailbone lifts up. Hands on hips, knees slightly less bent. Keep the stretch away from the back of knees. Hold for about three to five long, slow, complete inhalations and exhalations. Come up and repeat if you like.

▶ **Flexible**

Body is 90 degrees or more (horizontal or below) to the floor — ribs extend away from hips [Fig. 54]. Knees are straighter. Back is not rounded down but long, head in line with spine. Hands come down legs. If you're extremely flexible and you still don't feel a stretch in your hamstrings, move forward toward your toes a little (still keeping your heels on the floor). If your

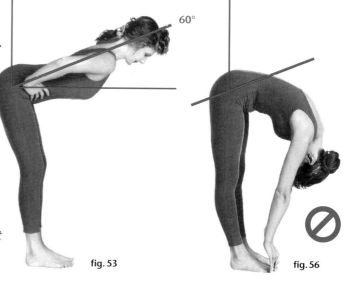

60°

fig. 53

fig. 56

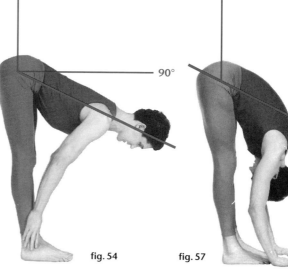

90°

fig. 54

fig. 57

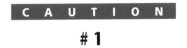

1

If you could not feel a stretch in your hamstrings (which is not at all unusual for new students), please turn now to "Variation for Hamstring Stretching" found in Appendix III.

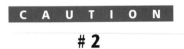

2

If you feel pain behind your knees, near the sitting bones in your buttocks, or in your lower back, do not push these exercises. Rather, always play the easier side of the stretch. If pain persists, slowly come out of the posture. Don't do this or any forward bending if you have a torn hamstring muscle.

hands reach the floor easily, then press them into the floor while bending the elbows inward toward the legs. Feel as if you are pushing the floor away from you while simultaneously lifting your sitting bones higher and your hamstrings will engage. Hold for about four to six long, slow, complete inhalations and exhalations. Come up and repeat if you have time.

Forward Bend Checklist

- Stand with your feet nearly parallel about two to three inches apart.
- Weight is balanced equally on both feet (forward and rear, left and right).
- Keep your spine long, maintaining your natural lumbar curve and rotate forward, not down.
- Go down only as far as you need to in order to feel the action (a stretch) in the center of your hamstring muscles, not the tendons behind your knees.
- Never bounce while doing stretching exercises.
- When coming up, initiate the rotation from your hips and pelvis, not from your shoulders.

Principle #3 Reviewed: Less Gets You More

*Once you learn how to move with proper alignment (by extending your body without traumatizing muscles, tendons, ligaments, or joints) **less when done correctly will always get you more.** This means by creating less aggression, effort, and pain, you will gain more flexibility, strength, endurance, and tone.*

Principle #6 Reviewed: Lengthening the Spine

Lengthening your spine lets you breathe more freely, enhances the stretch you feel, and helps your circulation and digestion. If you compress your spine, or slump, these processes become restricted.

Attitude Adjustment

I'm not going to give special attitude adjustment instructions for each exercise — usually you can just follow the arrows. Aggressive types, ease up by following upward arrows; if you tend to be more easygoing, follow the downward arrows, which makes the exercises more challenging. But since the standing Forward Bend is so basic to the ExTension program, I'd like you to go through some detailed adjustments:

▶ **Aggressive**

Remember, less always gets you more. Don't push your torso too low. Keep your knees bent. Start with the Tight example and practice for a couple of weeks until you feel your hamstrings and hips loosen up. Breathe and relax into the stretch and do not bounce.

▶ **Moderate**

Start with the example that's appropriate for your body type. Depending upon how comfortable that position is — and how ambitious and energetic you feel — challenge yourself to come down a little farther. Begin with bent knees, then experiment with straightening your legs a bit. Stop if you feel any pain behind your knees or in your back.

▶ **Easygoing**

Start with the example appropriate for your body type. Really pull your spine long and challenge yourself by bringing your torso as low as you can by lifting your sitting bones up without creating tightness behind your knees or in your lower back.

FINE-TUNING

"Deer Ears" — Imagine you are a deer, suddenly startled by a sound. Your ears will come up high above your shoulders, pulling your spine long. This increases the action in your hamstrings. That's how your head should be centered on your shoulders during the standing Forward Bend and most of the other exercises in this program [Fig.58, correct head]. Don't drop your head or lift your chin [Fig.59, incorrect head].

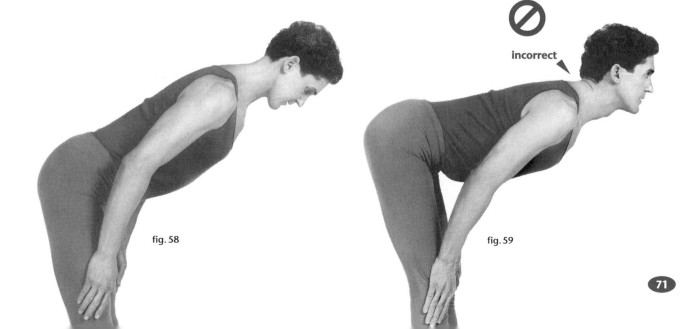

fig. 58

incorrect

fig. 59

Lunge

This adaptation of the "runner's lunge" will tone your thighs and enhance mobility of your hips and groin.

Start in Mountain pose. Then, bend your knees, fold over, and bring your hands all the way down to the floor, placing fingertips just outside of each foot, in line with your toes. [Fig. 60, transition to lunge]. Bend over as much as you need to in order to rest your ribs and belly on your thighs. Now, keep your fingertips on the floor directly underneath your shoulders, your index fingers parallel to each other and your fingers slightly spread to provide a solid base [Fig. 61, hand detail]. As soon as you feel securely anchored, place your left knee on the floor behind you and slide it back as far as you feel comfortable. Always keep your forward knee directly over its heel.

Keeping your left knee on the floor, extend your left leg gently behind you, without disturbing your right knee. This distance can be a little or a lot; so don't move quickly. You want to feel an easy stretch in your hip, groin, or thigh area. Check again to be sure that your right knee did not come forward of your right ankle (you should be able to look down and see the entire top of your foot). If you don't feel any "action" (stretch), extend your left leg farther back. If you feel too much "action" in your hip, groin, or thigh, move the rear knee closer to you.

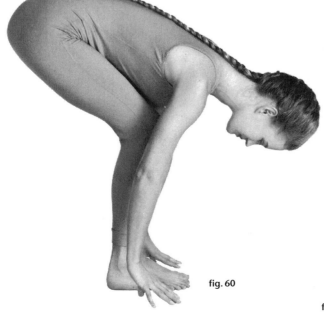

fig. 60

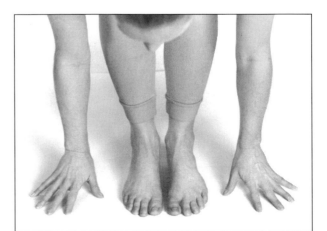

fig. 61

Try not to put a lot of weight directly on the kneecap of your rear leg. Instead, keep the weight always above the kneecap toward the bottom of your thigh.

▶ **_Tight_**
Your body placement will look like MJ with toes flexed [Fig.62] or toes extended [Fig.63]. You will be up on your fingertips. The more you practice this, the easier it becomes and the further your rear leg moves as your hips, groin, and thighs open up.

As long as your mechanics are correct, wherever you feel the action, whether it be in the hip, groin, or thigh, it is appropriate for your body. As you pull your spine longer (this feels as if you are stretching your belly), you'll feel an increased action in your hips, groin, or thighs (this is a proof of Principle #6). What you want to avoid is discomfort in your hips, thighs, or groin, or tightness in your back. If you feel as though your wrists are getting mashed, read "Fine-Tuning" on page 75.

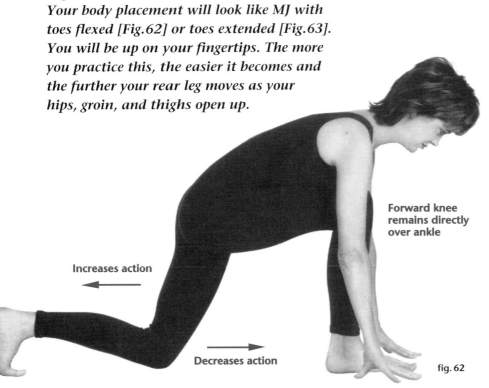

Forward knee remains directly over ankle

Increases action

Decreases action

fig. 62

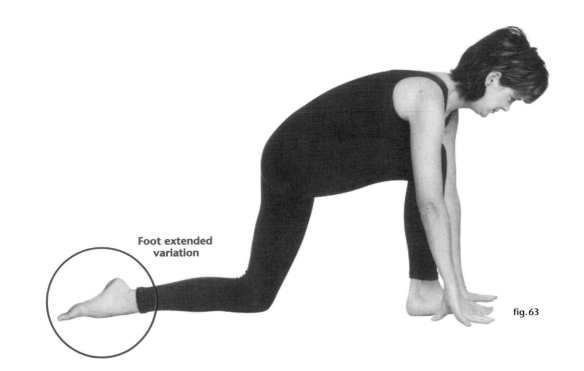

Foot extended variation

fig. 63

Lunge

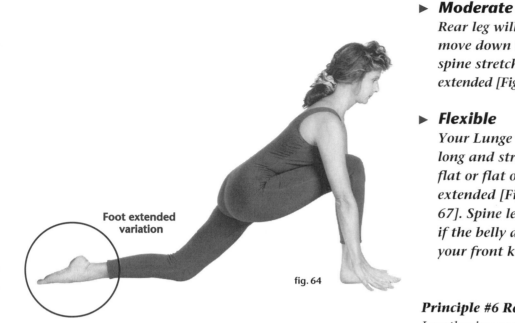

Foot extended variation

fig. 64

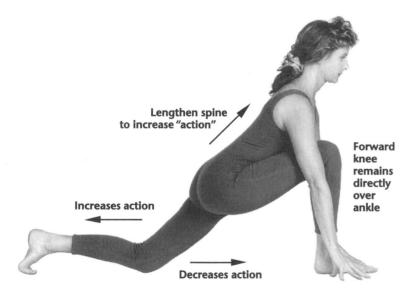

Lengthen spine to increase "action"

Increases action

Decreases action

Forward knee remains directly over ankle

fig. 65

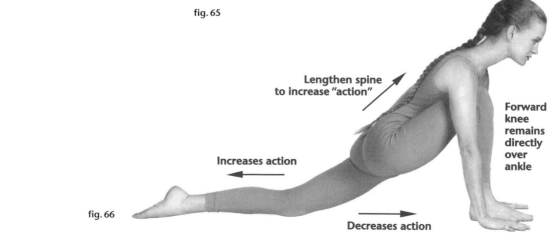

Lengthen spine to increase "action"

Increases action

Decreases action

Forward knee remains directly over ankle

fig. 66

▶ **Moderate**

Rear leg will stretch out further. Hands move down toward the floor, neck and spine stretch long. Toes may be either extended [Fig.64] or curled under [Fig.65].

▶ **Flexible**

Your Lunge will be deeper, rear leg very long and stretched out. Hands almost flat or flat on floor. Toes may be extended [Fig.66] or curled under [Fig. 67]. Spine lengthens so that you feel as if the belly and ribs move farther toward your front knee.

Principle #6 Reviewed

Lengthening your spine lets you breathe more freely, enhances the stretch you feel, and helps your circulation and digestion. If you compress your spine, or slump, these processes become restricted.

It's important to keep your head in line with your spine by keeping your chin in a neutral position. Don't lift or drop your chin; instead, think and do Deer Ears as presented in "Fine-Tuning" on page 71. As you extend your spine long, think about extending through both the top of your head and the bottom of your spine (but keep your rear knee on the floor). And don't forget to breathe.

FINE-TUNING

Whenever your hands are on the floor, check the position of your hands and fingers. Keep your index fingers parallel to each other and the rest of your hand turned out as in Figure 68, correct hand placement. Otherwise, you will compress your wrists [Fig.69, incorrect hand placement]. As a beginner, stay up on your fingertips. Then adjust toward Moderate or Flexible by gradually flattening your hands, or by extending your rear leg away from you, or both.

C A U T I O N

You may get a foot cramp in the Lunge position. Muscle cramping is an involuntary reflex usually caused by tight muscle or fascial tissue and almost always lessens with regular practice. But for now, if you do cramp, simply change the position of your foot (or other body part). If that doesn't seem to work, lie down and do the Three-Part Breath. If you regularly cramp while doing these exercises, try drinking some water before you practice. If cramping continues to be chronic and painful (sometimes a sign of nutritional deficiency), you might want to consult a physician or nutritionist.

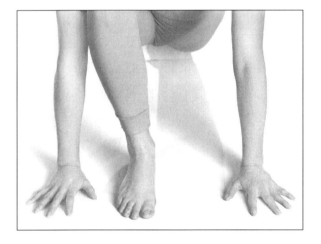

fig. 68

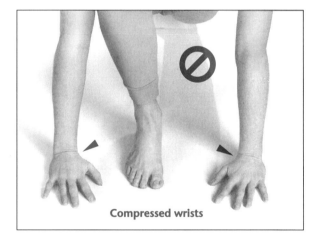

Compressed wrists

fig. 69

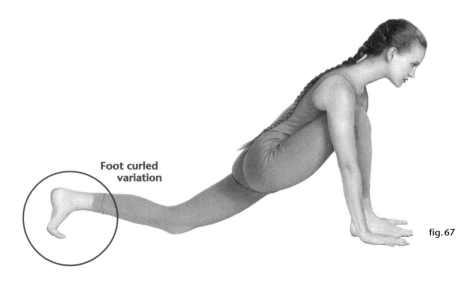

Foot curled variation

fig. 67

Plank Position

The Plank and Plank Variation are powerful all-over strengtheners for your arms and shoulders. Done regularly, they will really firm up your arms and chest.

Start in the Lunge Position with your left leg back. Now, keeping your hands in place (your hands are turned outward with index fingers parallel to each other), activate (as you learned in the introduction) and flatten them firmly on the floor. Now move your right knee back so it's in line with your left. Curl your toes under your feet. Then, come up on your toes, straighten

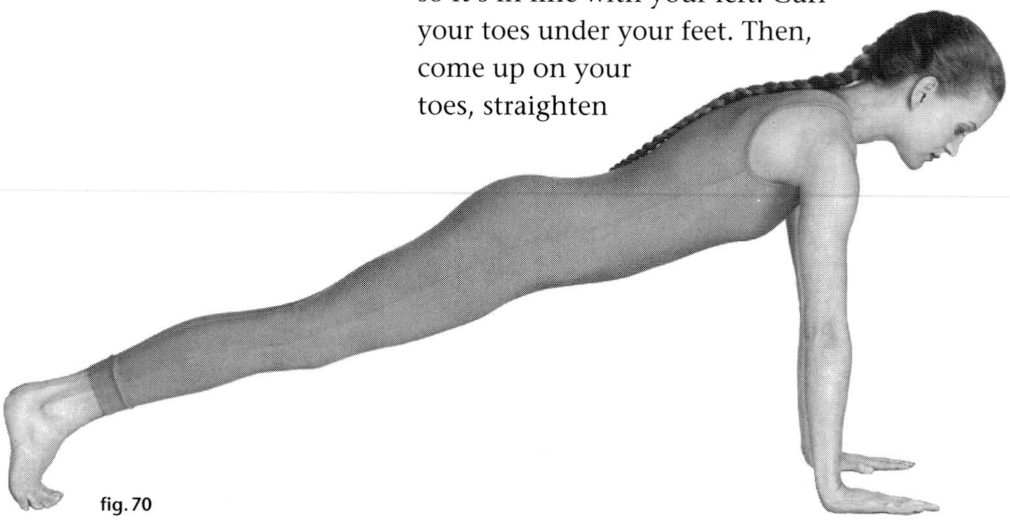

fig. 70

(but don't lock) your elbows, and stretch your spine long [Fig. 70]. You'll be in a "push-up position" balancing on your hands and your

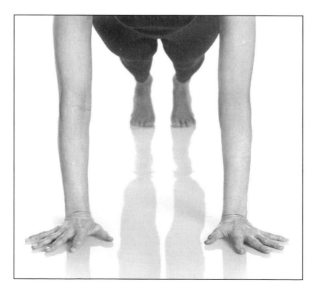

fig. 71

toes. This is the Plank position.

Make sure that your hands are directly under your shoulders. Rotate your elbows in or out so that, if there were headlights positioned on the inside of each elbow, those headlights would intersect about two and a half to three feet in front of you [Fig.71].

To lengthen your spine, press your hands strongly into the floor and feel as if you are lifting your chest up through your shoulder blades, while extending your heels away from your Deer Ears (a long, extended neck).

Keep your buttocks in line with your spine, as a "plank," so there's one smooth line from your head to your feet with no sinking down [Fig.72] or jackknifing up [Fig.73]. It may help to look sideways in a mirror the first few times. Now, just hold the position and breathe for one to three deep breaths. Make sure your

Pelvis has dropped

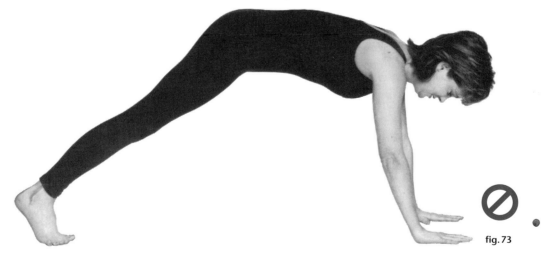

fig.72

Pelvis has lifted up

fig.73

CAUTION

If you've recently had
abdominal surgery, practice the
Plank without the variation.

WHAT YOU'LL FEEL

*You'll experience an
opening of your chest and
toning of your arms. You'll
also notice that the posture
guides you toward align-
ment by compelling you to
pull your spine long. When
you add the variation,
keeping your elbows
moving inward, you'll feel
the action in your triceps
(upper rear arms), chest,
and abdominal muscles.
You shouldn't feel tightness
in your lower back or neck;
if you do, check your form
in a mirror.*

chest is lifted, your head is in line with your
spine (it helps to look straight down at the
floor beneath you) and your wrists aren't
feeling mashed. If they are, it means either
that you're not lifting through your shoulders
and upper back or your hands are improperly
positioned [Fig. 74, incorrect hand position].

From the Plank, you can do a few modified
push-ups for upper body, arm, and stomach
strengthening. (I call this exercise the Plank
Variation.) Bend and lower both knees to the
floor (beginners can lower one at a time)
keeping your hands in place [Fig. 75]. Dorsiflex
your feet (that's pointing your heel away from
you) and bend your lower legs up. Then, while
slowly inhaling, bend your elbows (always
keeping them *close* to your sides) and slowly
lower your body any amount toward the floor
[Fig. 76]. You may go down as little or as far as
you like, as long as you can go down and come
up with a straight back. Slowly push back up
as you exhale, keeping your elbows close to
your sides.

Don't allow your body to sink down
[Fig. 77]. Begin with one to three repetitions,
always keeping your spine straight. As your
strength develops, increase your repetitions.

When you're ready, simply lower both feet
to the floor (one at a time) and relax on your
hands and knees for a moment, breathing
deeply, softly, and smoothly.

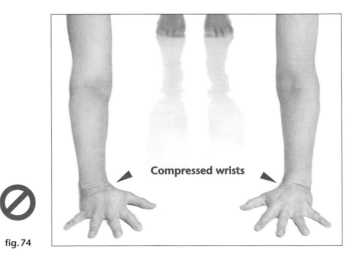

fig. 74

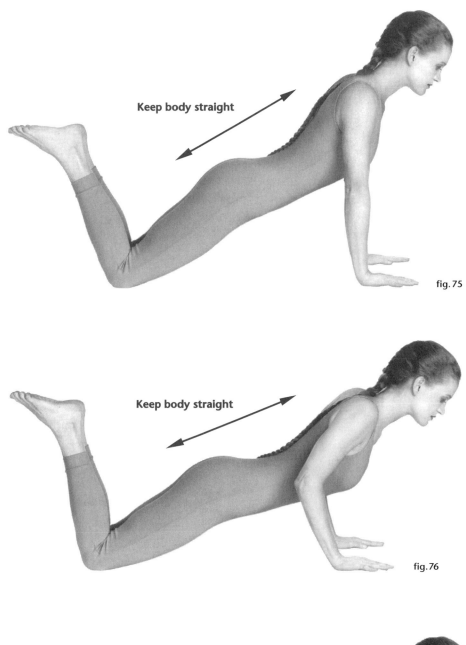

Keep body straight

fig. 75

Keep body straight

fig. 76

FINE-TUNING

*While pushing up during the Plank Variation, feel as if you are "sucking up your belly" as you exhale and you will notice that coming up becomes easier. Once you can easily do a number of them, practice the advanced Plank Variation by **not** bending your knees:*

Keep your body, all the way from your heels to your head, as straight as a board, while going up and down. Remember to inhale going down and exhale coming up always keeping your elbows to the sides of your body. If you feel your body collapsing, just go back to the regular Plank Variation until you develop more strength.

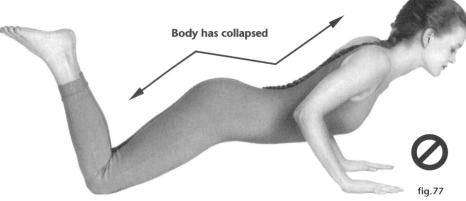

Body has collapsed

fig. 77

Pose of the Child

Although it appears to be a simple exercise, Pose of the Child is quite important. It reinforces proper hand foundations. It helps release back tension and it enhances breathing by teaching you how to extend your spine and neck.

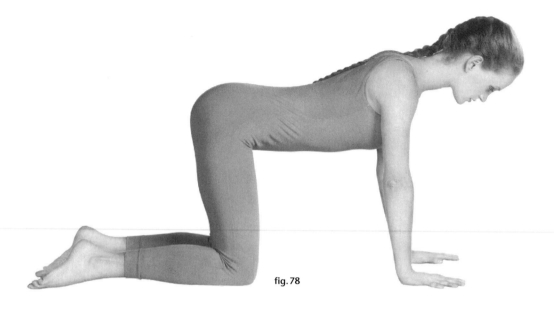

fig. 78

Begin on your hands and knees. Put your hands on the floor right underneath your shoulders, your knees directly under your hips [Fig.78]. Use the same hand and arm positioning as with the Plank, active hands, with your index fingers parallel to each other and both hands turned slightly out (if necessary, refer back to Figure 71, page 76). Also press down through the four points of your hands (they're actually the same as those on your feet): the inner and outer heels of your hands and the inner and outer balls of your

Inner heel

Inner ball

Outer heel   Outer ball

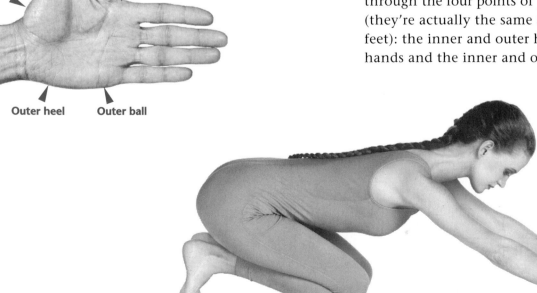

fig. 80

hands [Fig. 79]. Make any adjustments to your hands and arms now because it will be very important to keep them in place through the coming exercises.

Once your hands are in place, sit back on your heels. You may need to adjust your knee position, drawing closer to or farther away from your hands, to make yourself more comfortable. You can curl your toes under or extend them and rest on the top of your feet, whichever feels better [Figs. 80 and 81].

Now, keeping your hands active and securely pressing down (especially the inner ball mounts) on the floor, lift your chest while gently pulling your belly forward toward your knees. Keep your inner elbows turned upward, not downward, shoulders moving away from your ears and shoulder blades wide. Your neck elongates (see "Fine-Tuning"). It's almost as if you're pulling the floor toward you as your torso moves forward.

Take a few long, deep breaths, pull your spine even longer, keep your shoulders wide, and pull your rib cage forward but do not allow your hands to move. When you do this correctly, you'll feel your belly gently stretching.

C A U T I O N

If you have any knee pain, sit up, place a thin, tightly rolled wash towel snugly behind the painful knee (or both if necessary) and deep into the joint. If you are pregnant or have a large stomach, you should widen your knees to make room for your belly.

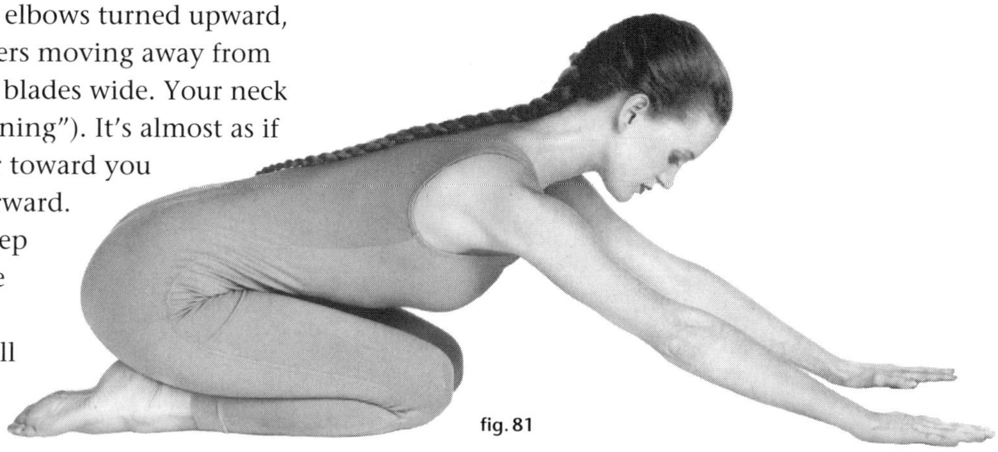

fig. 81

▶ **Tight**

Generally, the tighter you are, the higher your upper body will be from your thighs and the farther your buttocks will be from your heels [Fig. 82]. Hold this pose for

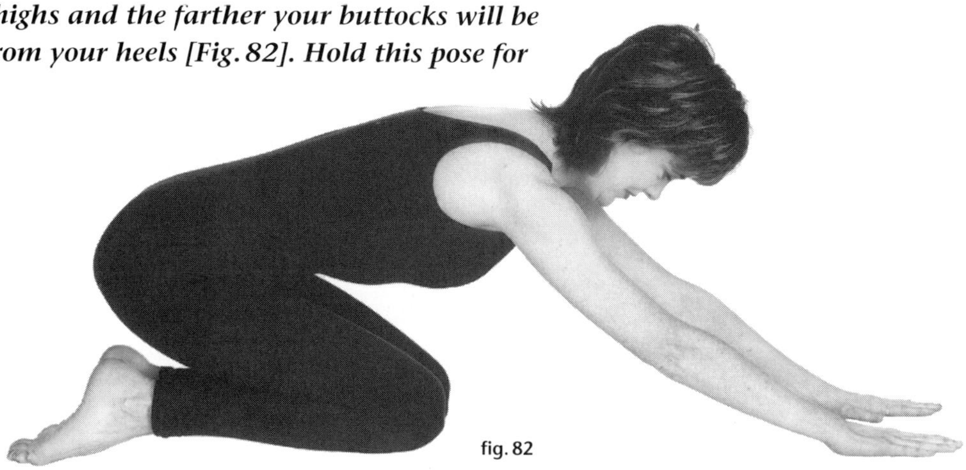

fig. 82

three to six breaths, longer if you can, but not if it causes pain, which will cause further tightness. If your ankles hurt, put a tightly rolled towel directly under both ankles and then reassume the pose. If you feel any knee discomfort, refer to the "Caution." To reduce overall discomfort, draw your hands closer to your knees, lift your torso higher and then reactivate your hands. Your toes may be extended or curled under your feet.

▶ Moderate and Flexible

Moderate [Fig. 81] and Flexible [Fig. 83] are similar. The more flexible you are, the closer your chest will come to your thighs and the closer your buttocks will be to your heels. Keep your torso and neck extending with every exhalation. Keep your hands "glued" to the floor while "pulling" your hands toward you to help extend your spine. Toes may be extended or curled under feet.

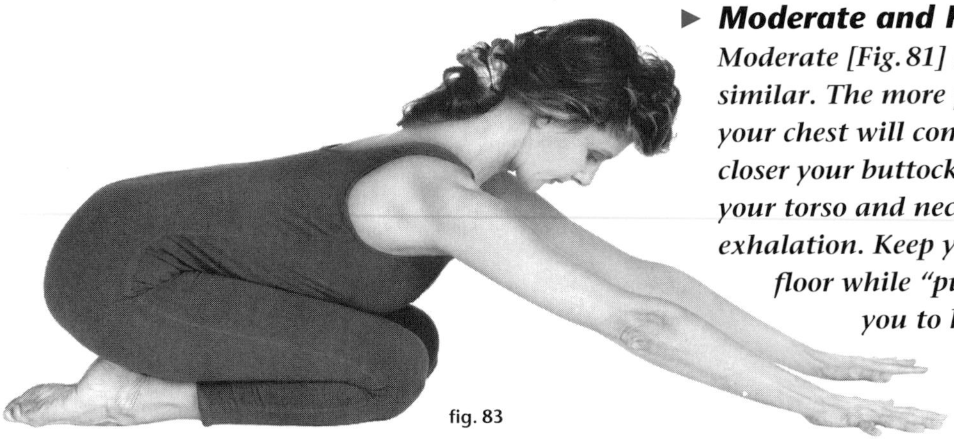

fig. 83

Attitude Adjustment

▶ Aggressive

Don't try to push buttocks to heels if you have any knee or hip pain. If you experience any pain in this posture, use the props as suggested above. Relax your neck and jaw. Move your hands a little closer to you and let this stretch feel good. Don't hurry it.

▶ Moderate and Easygoing

Don't get too comfortable in this pose. If you can bring your buttocks closer to your heels and your upper body closer to your thighs, do it, as long as you stop before you feel pain, and keep breathing. Keep extending your spine long, and keep your hands and arms active.

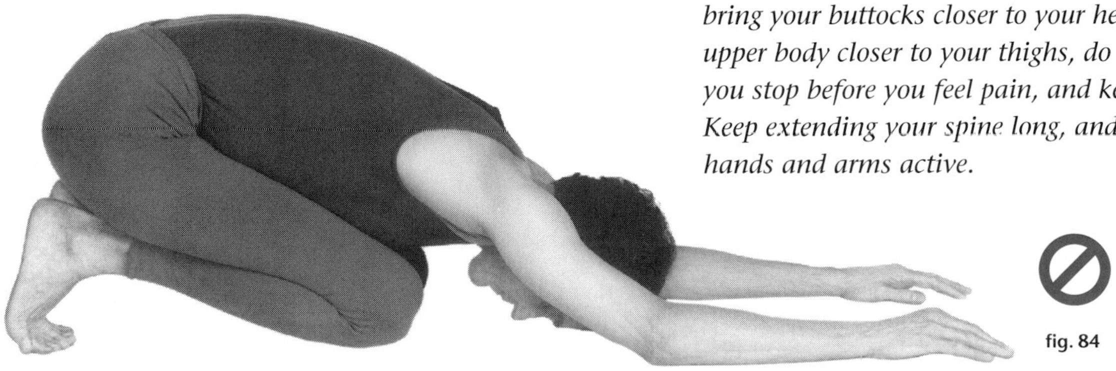

fig. 84

Before we move on, let's do another experiment. While in Pose of the Child, put your head down on the floor [Fig.84]. Notice how your neck and shoulders immediately constrict and how your breathing constricts as well. Then lift your head back up into alignment with your spine (Deer Ears) and again broaden your shoulders. How does this feel? Go back and forth a couple of times and compare how much better you feel when your head is up (don't forget to widen your shoulders) than when your head is down.

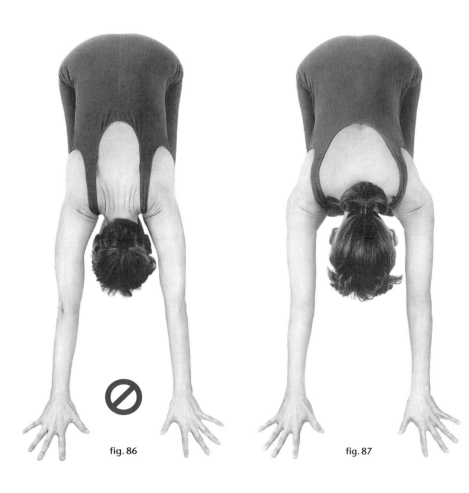

fig. 85

fig. 86

fig. 87

FINE-TUNING

While broadening your shoulders, think about drawing your neck and spine long — into your Deer Ears mode — simultaneously pulling your hips and tailbone away from your hands. Figure 85 shows Sam helping Annie lengthen her neck to create a longer spine.

Here's a way to visualize the widening of your shoulders in this pose: think of your armpits rotating inward, then bringing your lats (the muscles just underneath them and to the sides of your body) down and toward your chest. Inhale and while keeping your hands actively pulling toward you, widen your shoulder blades as you exhale. Figure 86 shows Susan from above in Pose of the Child with her shoulders scrunched while Figure 87 shows her with wide shoulder blades. Which one looks more comfortable?

Cobra

This is one of the most misunderstood of all exercises. Cobra is really a spine extender, not a "back bend" as generally thought. Practiced correctly, it will tone your belly and strengthen and tone the back of your arms.

The cobra is not for everyone. If you are three months pregnant or more or have recently had abdominal or chest surgery, go from Pose of the Child directly to the Cat/Cow Stretch. If you have back problems, consult your doctor.

The first time or two that you try the Cobra, do the Tight adaptation as shown by MJ, even if you are Moderate to Flexible. Then proceed according to your body type.

The Cobra can begin from Pose of the Child, or you can start from your hands and knees. Maintaining your hand position, lower your elbows to the floor [Fig. 88A] (see page 86) and slide out your legs one at a time [Fig. 88B] or both together, if you prefer, ending up on your belly [Fig. 88C]. Be sure that when you look down, your elbows are on the floor forward of your shoulders. Your hands, wrists, and elbows should still be parallel to — and only as wide as — your shoulders. Keep your hands active: index fingers parallel, thumbs and fingers spread.

Now, press your hands down (especially the inner and outer ball mounts) strongly into the floor and do not allow them to slide toward you as you raise your head and your chest slowly off the floor *pulling* your torso forward. Your elbows might even come off the floor but if they do, *always keep them bent.* If your back hurts even the slightest amount, keep your elbows on the floor. As you lift, *pull your rib cage forward.* Your belly will follow and you should feel a stretching there as you pull forward. Use your triceps (the back of your arms) to *pull* the floor toward you. It's almost as if you were lying on the floor facing a wall and you were trying to pull your belly up the wall by using only your hands. This helps your spine lengthen.

Do not arch your head back but keep it aligned with your spine by lengthening through the top of your head as in Deer Ears.

Tighten your buttocks and keep your pelvis on the floor to help support your lower back as you hold this pose. Also keep your elbows bent. Breathe deeply, and as you continue to pull your chest and rib cage forward, you'll feel the stretch in your belly and an action in your triceps. Relax your jaw and keep your face soft.

Repeat two to four times breathing deeply, smoothly, and quietly throughout. When you're ready, keep your hands in place and slowly let yourself come forward and down to the floor. Do not drop out of the Cobra. Relax for a few deep breaths.

WHAT YOU'LL FEEL

When you're in the Cobra position, with your buttocks tight, you should feel a stretch in your belly and perhaps across your chest and a lengthening of your spine. Done correctly, the triceps are activated (see detail, Fig. 89), the Cobra is a powerful toner and strengthener for your upper arms (a flabby area for many people over 40) and your back. By pulling forward, you will avoid a feeling of compressing your lower back. By keeping your head in a neutral position (Deer Ears), you avoid constricting your neck and overstretching your throat.

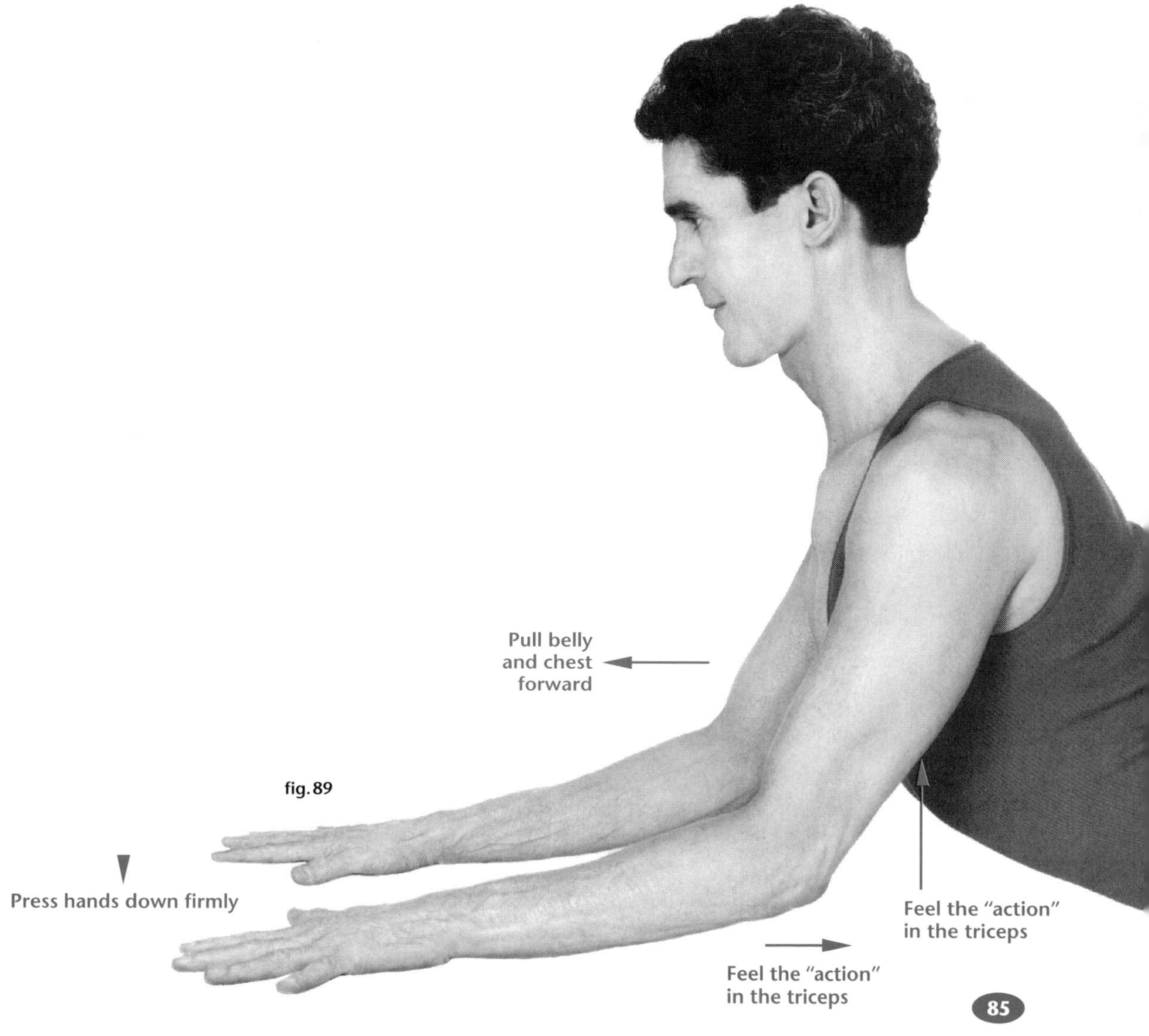

Pull belly and chest forward

fig. 89

Press hands down firmly

Feel the "action" in the triceps

Feel the "action" in the triceps

► *Tight*

For transition from Pose of the Child, place elbows on the floor [Fig. 88A] and slide back one leg at a time [Fig. 88B] behind you. In the Cobra, elbows must remain forward of shoulders and on the floor. Pull belly forward and chest up only a slight amount [Fig. 88C]. If you experience any back pain at all, move your elbows forward an inch or two at a time until you can come up without pain.

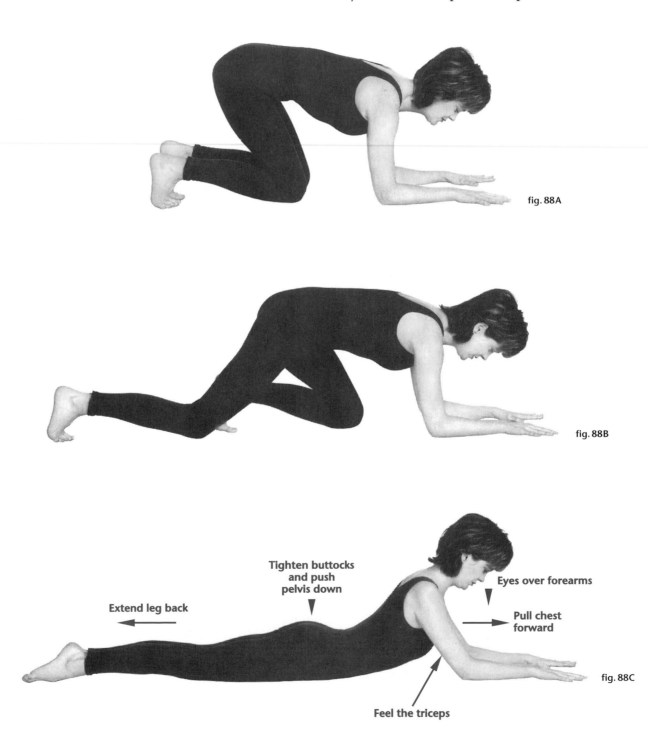

fig. 88A

fig. 88B

Tighten buttocks and push pelvis down

Eyes over forearms

Extend leg back

Pull chest forward

Feel the triceps

fig. 88C

▶ *Moderate*

For transition from Pose of the Child [Fig. 90A], place elbows on floor and slide both legs behind you [Fig. 90B] in a smooth, continuous motion. Eyes will be over your wrists; hands will end up well forward of shoulders, elbows close to sides. Elbows stay bent and come off the floor slightly [Fig. 90C]. If you experience any back pain at all, move your hands forward by an inch or two until there is no back pain.

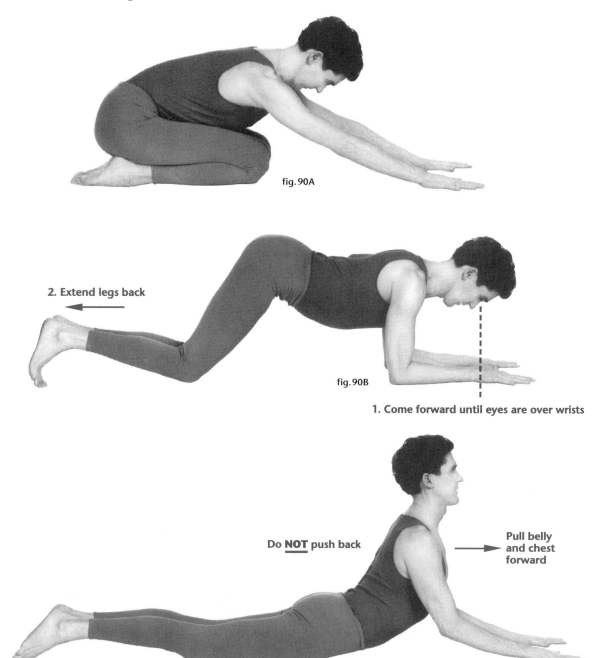

fig. 90A

2. Extend legs back

fig. 90B

1. Come forward until eyes are over wrists

Do NOT push back

Pull belly and chest forward

fig. 90C

▶ **Flexible**

For transition from hands and knees, simultaneously lower elbows, bringing your chin close to the floor with eyes directly over fingertips [Fig. 91A] and slide both legs back behind you in a smooth, continuous motion [Fig. 91B]. Pull forward and up as far as you comfortably can. Hands will be under or slightly forward of the shoulders (or, if you are extremely flexible, slightly behind the shoulders) with elbows moving in close to the sides of your body. Elbows can come off the floor, but remember to always keep them bent as you pull your belly forward [Fig. 91C].

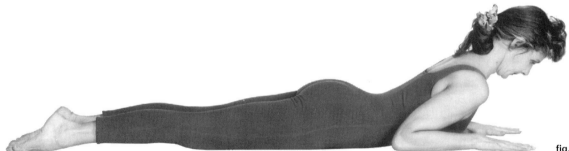

2. Slide legs back

1. Come forward until eyes are over fingertips

fig. 91A

fig. 91B

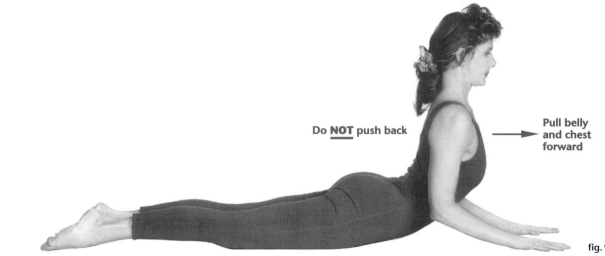

Do **NOT** push back

Pull belly and chest forward

fig. 91C

Attitude Adjustment

▶ *Aggressive*

Don't be tempted to push back when you're in the completed Cobra. Instead, always pull forward and never come up higher than you comfortably can. Remember that less will always get you more. Avoid any back pain. Even just a little. Do several rounds of the Cobra but do not be in a hurry. Instead, experiment with how slowly you can come up and down, inhaling while you come up and exhaling while you come down.

▶ *Moderate*

If you feel like challenging yourself more, and as long as you do not create any back pain, pull on the floor more assertively, which further activates your triceps and may bring your elbows up. Don't be concerned about how high you can bring your body but how far forward you can pull your chest and belly.

▶ *Easygoing*

Challenge yourself by pulling the floor a little harder (keeping your elbows bent). Feel it in your triceps, but avoid any back pain. Hold for longer periods of time, deep breathing throughout. Your triceps will probably become a little sore, but if you practice continually, the soreness will quickly go away.

C A U T I O N

If you experience any back pain at all, regardless of your flexibility, always move your hands farther forward until you can do the exercise with no back pain at all. Be certain to maintain triceps action throughout. If you still feel some pain, stop.

Cat/Cow Stretch

The Cat/Cow Stretch is an optional exercise, not usually included in the complete Sun Salutation. But it helps teach you a crucial movement for the following pose — Downward Facing Dog. The Cat/Cow can also be done on its own to relieve back or hip stiffness.

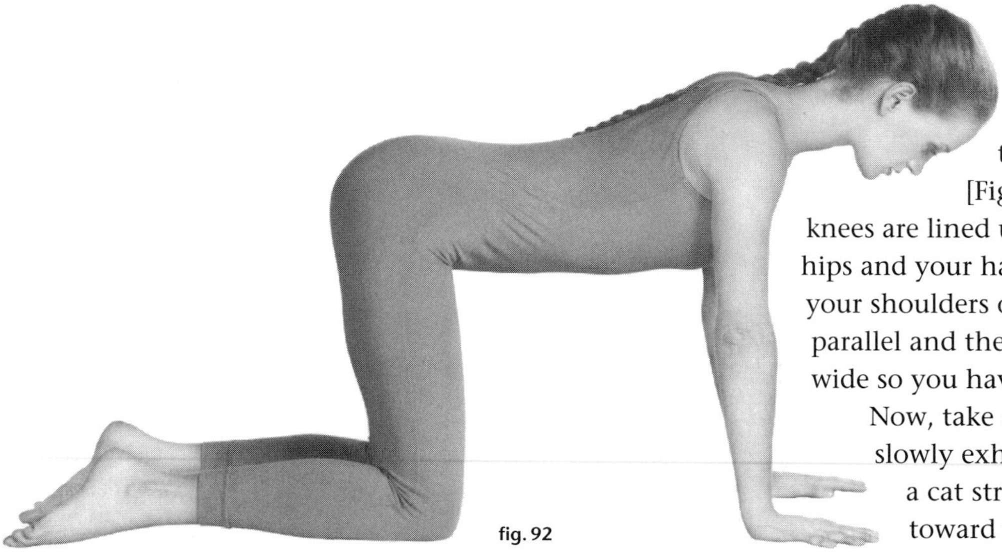

fig. 92

From the Cobra, go to your hands and knees [Fig. 92]. Check that your knees are lined up just underneath your hips and your hands are directly under your shoulders on the floor, index fingers parallel and the rest of your fingers fairly wide so you have a firm base.

Now, take a deep breath, and as you slowly exhale, imagine that you're a cat stretching your back up toward the ceiling. As you relax your head down, bring your belly up so that it becomes concave and your spine is rounded up toward the ceiling as far as is comfortable for you. This is the Cat stretch [Fig. 93].

Next, inhaling through your nose (if you can), lift your head and your tail up toward the ceiling while you drop your belly down. Your back will now be curving slightly, which means a slight arching of your back. This is the Cow stretch. It should be a smooth movement, done by simply tilting your buttocks up, but not overarching your back [Fig. 94].

Remember this sensation of lifting your buttocks but not overarching your back — it helps you learn the Downward Facing Dog pose, which follows. If you feel any discomfort in your neck, don't take your head as high as Annie has done in Figure 94.

Now, as you exhale, do the Cat stretch, arching your back up; inhale and do the Cow stretch, dropping your belly down. Go back and forth slowly a few times. Keep your elbows lengthening the entire time and keep your breathing deep, long, and smooth throughout. Do about six to eight rounds and when you're ready to stop, stay on your hands and knees breathing easily, or go back and rest in Pose of the Child.

► **All Body Types**

Do not be overly aggressive in either the Cat or the Cow. Always remember to coordinate your breathing with your movements and to keep your elbows lengthening throughout.

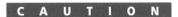

C A U T I O N

While doing the cow stretch, don't overarch your head back, and don't push either stretch into pain. If you have back problems, consult your doctor before doing this stretch.

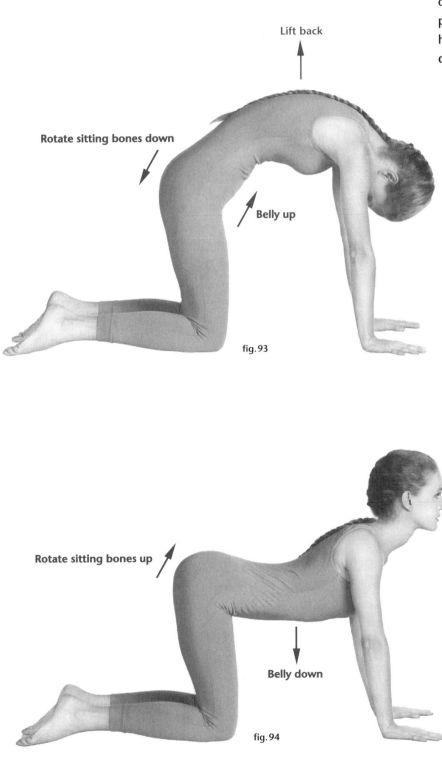

Lift back

Rotate sitting bones down

Belly up

fig. 93

Rotate sitting bones up

Belly down

fig. 94

WHAT YOU'LL FEEL

This is a wonderful stretch for your entire back, especially your lower back. As you arch up into the Cat position, you'll probably feel a stretch across your upper back and shoulders and a tightening of your abdominal muscles. When you curve down into the Cow position, the muscles along your spine and in your neck should feel long, not compressed, and your stomach muscles may pull gently. If you feel any discomfort in your lower back during the Cow, don't arch as much.

Downward Facing Dog

The Downward Facing Dog is one of the best yoga-based exercises you can do. *It promotes a true balance between flexibility and strength. And when done well, it's a beautiful pose. But unless you really pay attention to the following instructions, the Down Dog (its nickname) can be a difficult pose to learn. So I'm going to introduce the pose using props like a chair or a step, and I want you — regardless of your flexibility — to begin here. Once you learn the basics and feel what you're supposed to feel in the stretch, the most flexible of you will get down on the floor almost immediately, but please try it this way first.*

The object of the Downward Facing Dog is to feel an isolated stretch in your hamstrings while you are lengthening your spine and keeping your neck and shoulders tension-free.

Place a chair securely against a wall (or you can use the first two or three steps of a staircase). Kneel in front of it and put your

fig. 95

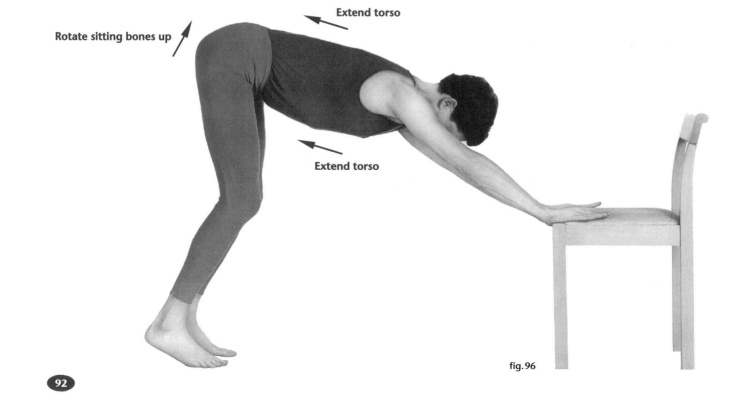

Rotate sitting bones up

Extend torso

Extend torso

fig. 96

palms flat on the front edge surface, about
shoulder width apart, your hands rotated out
so that the index fingers are parallel and your
wrists and arms are *straight*. Press down on the
four points of both hands: the inner and outer
ball mounts and the inner and outer heels.
(Your hands and arms are placed exactly as
you learned in Pose of the Child as Susan
shows in Figure 95.)

Come up on your tiptoes and lift your
hips toward the ceiling by lengthening your
legs, but *keep your knees bent* and your heels up
high [Fig. 96]. Put your head into a neutral
position (not lifting up or dropping down) so
that you can broaden your shoulder blades
and lengthen your spine. Make sure your back
doesn't round up or that your head doesn't
drop down [Fig. 97, incorrect Dog pose]. Your
body will look roughly like a upside down "V"
but with slightly bent knees.

Now, take a breath and as you let it out,
widen your shoulders, just as you did in Pose
of the Child [Fig. 95], imagining the muscles
just under your armpits (your lats) widening

NOTE TO THE VERY FLEXIBLE

*If you're a very flexible
person, it may be difficult
for you to feel a hamstring
stretch while you do this
with you hands on a chair
or step (although you
probably will when your
spine lengthens, your
shoulders widen, and your
sitting bones rotate up). Just
let your knees to go come
down toward the floor,
paying particular attention
to all the other details.*

*If you still haven't
felt an isolated hamstring
stretch, then start with
your hands on the floor;
again, adhering to the
details as given.*

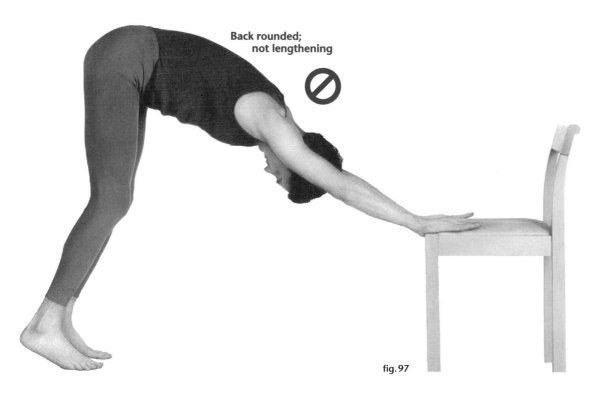

Back rounded;
not lengthening

fig. 97

WHAT YOU'LL FEEL

If you're doing the Downward Facing Dog correctly, you'll feel a primary stretch in the center of your hamstrings. You should also feel a broadening of your shoulders and a lengthening and opening of your chest. Everything should feel long — your torso, your abdomen, your spine, your arms, your legs, your neck — and expanded. If you feel any pain or discomfort behind your knees, bend your knees a little more, or lift your heels a little higher, or both. Let up on the posture.

Downward Facing Dog pose will become a fabulous exercise, and, although you will always feel challenged by it, the pose will ultimately become one of your most balanced and comfortable exercises.

out the sides of your back. Keep them down and wide [Fig. 98, shoulders open and wide], not crunched [Fig. 99, shoulders scrunched].

Lift your chest, don't let it drop down, and breathe easily.

Next, rotate your tailbone up, *just as you did in the Cow stretch.* Think back to the Forward Bend and the duck's tail that you want to lift up and show off. (If you need to review how that feels, turn back to page 90 and do it again now.) Keeping your knees bent, your head in alignment with your torso (Deer Ears), and your palms nailed to the floor, extend your hips away from your hands — reach them high toward the wall behind you — to lengthen your spine even more. You should now feel your hamstrings stretch.

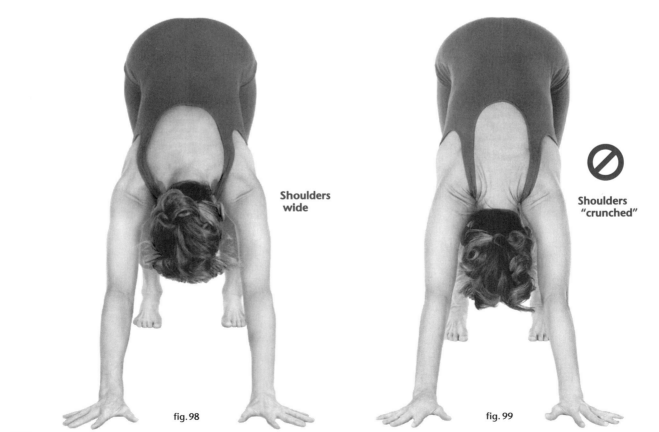

Shoulders wide

Shoulders "crunched"

fig. 98

fig. 99

After you've clearly felt that isolated hamstring stretch while you have your hands up on a chair or step, it's time to go a little lower. You can use a bench [Fig.100], equal stacks of books supporting each hand about 9 to 12 inches off the floor, or a lower step if you are using stairs. Details are the same as above.

And once you've really isolated the stretch again, using the lower step or books, you can start with your hands on the floor.

The instructions are still pretty much the same, except you start on your hands and knees (the Cat/Cow position) with your hands right under your shoulders and your knees directly under your hips (make sure your hands are anchored and active) [Fig.101], curl your toes under your feet, and, again, come up on your tiptoes by lifting your hips toward the ceiling and keeping your knees bent slightly throughout. Your body will come closer to being an inverted "V."

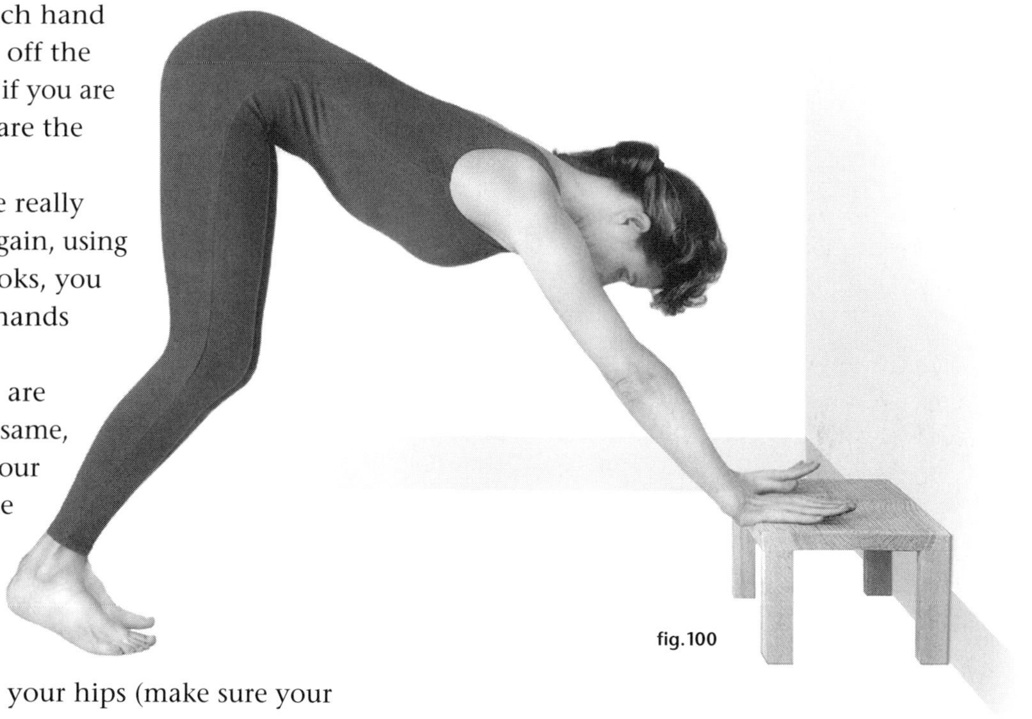

fig.100

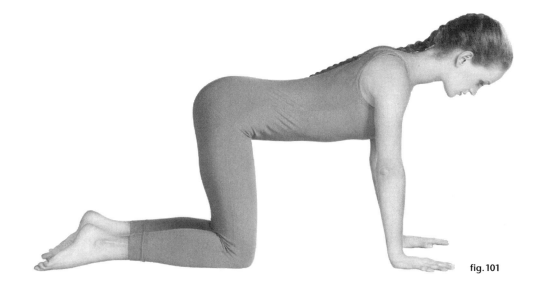

fig.101

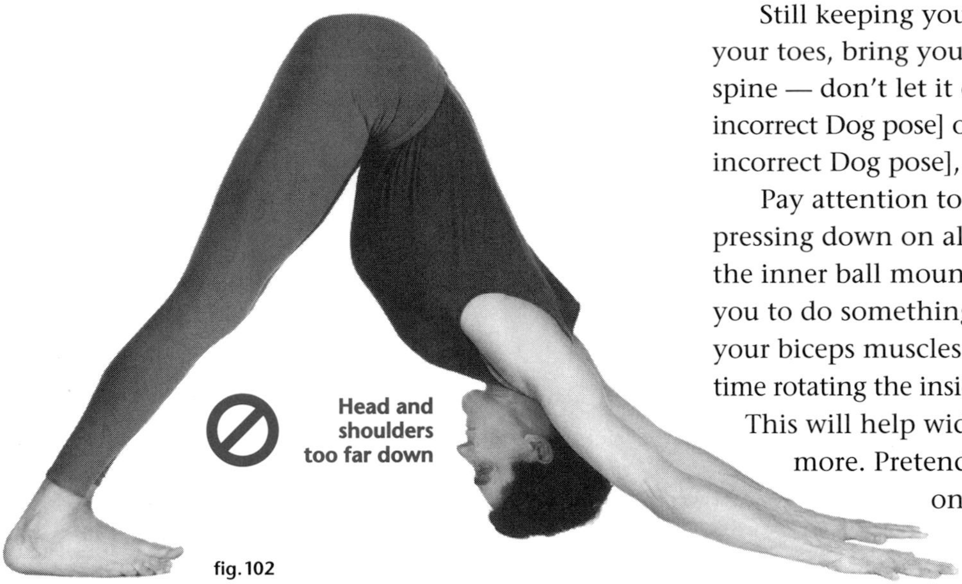

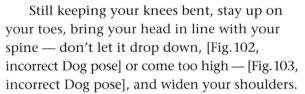

Head and shoulders too far down

fig. 102

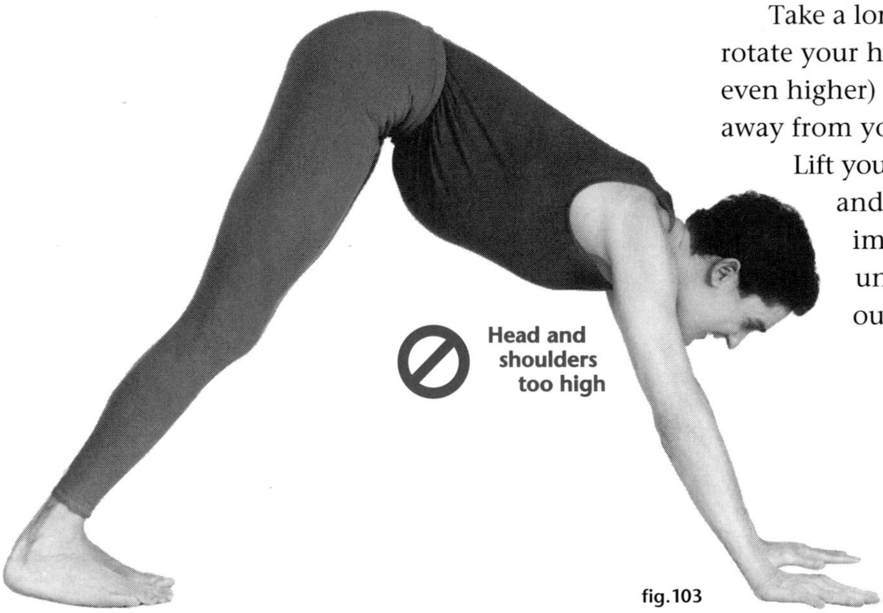

Head and shoulders too high

fig. 103

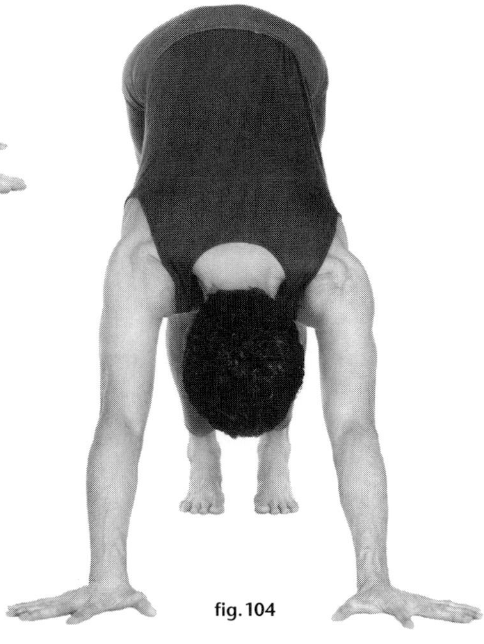

Still keeping your knees bent, stay up on your toes, bring your head in line with your spine — don't let it drop down, [Fig. 102, incorrect Dog pose] or come too high — [Fig. 103, incorrect Dog pose], and widen your shoulders.

Pay attention to your hands. Keep them pressing down on all four points, especially the inner ball mounts. Next, I'm going to ask you to do something difficult. Can you rotate your biceps muscles upward while at the same time rotating the inside of your wrists downward? This will help widen your shoulders even more. Pretend that there are headlights on the inside of each elbow and you want to rotate them so that the beams from the headlights will intersect about two to three feet in front of you [Fig. 104].

Take a long, deep breath, and as you exhale, rotate your hips (by lifting your duck feathers even higher) and extend your hips even farther away from your hands, lengthening your spine. Lift your chest up, don't drop it down, and widen your shoulders even more, imagining that the muscles just under your armpits are "puffing" out through your armpits.

fig. 104

▶ *Tight*

Don't start with your hands on the floor unless you clearly feel your hamstrings stretching. Otherwise, use a prop. Knees remain significantly bent, heels high off the floor [Fig.105].

Check that your feet are parallel, about six to eight inches apart. Hold for two to four long deep, smooth, quiet breaths. Feel as if you are lengthening your spine on every exhalation. Come down onto your hands and knees and rest. Repeat three to six times.

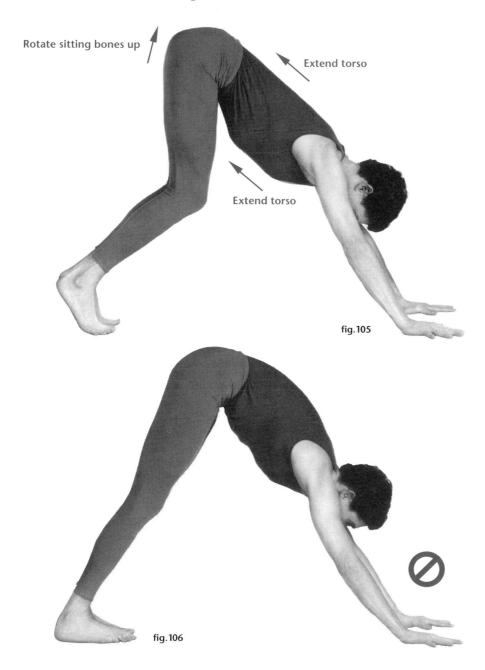

Rotate sitting bones up

Extend torso

Extend torso

fig.105

fig.106

C A U T I O N

For Tight and Moderate:
Unless you have very flexible hamstrings, you run the risk of irritating or injuring your lower back if you straighten your knees in Downward Facing Dog. Look at Figure 106. Here I demonstrate average to tight flexibility. Notice what happens to my lower back when I straighten my legs; my back is rounded and its tissues are overstretched and strained. If you have a tendency toward lower back dysfunction, this could exacerbate your condition (and usually does). Look at the Tight and Moderate Figures 105 and 107. Notice that regardless of flexibility, the back remains long by bending the knees. Unless you are *very* supple in your hamstrings, keep your knees bent while isolating your hamstring stretches.

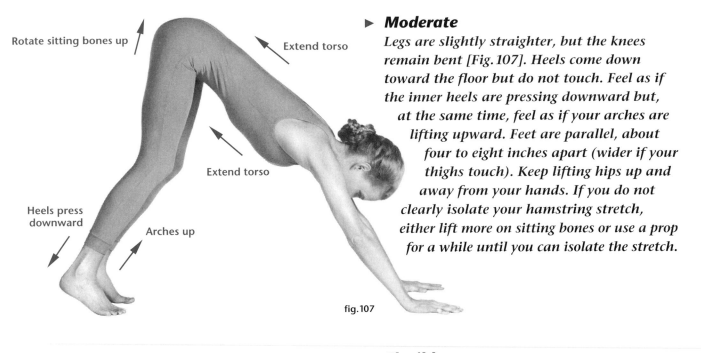

Rotate sitting bones up

Extend torso

Extend torso

Heels press downward

Arches up

fig. 107

▶ Moderate

Legs are slightly straighter, but the knees remain bent [Fig. 107]. Heels come down toward the floor but do not touch. Feel as if the inner heels are pressing downward but, at the same time, feel as if your arches are lifting upward. Feet are parallel, about four to eight inches apart (wider if your thighs touch). Keep lifting hips up and away from your hands. If you do not clearly isolate your hamstring stretch, either lift more on sitting bones or use a prop for a while until you can isolate the stretch.

▶ Flexible

Knees might be totally straight but probably bent just a little [Fig. 108]. Inside of heels move downward to the floor while inner arches of the feet lift up. Create a feeling that the inner knees press toward each other, but do not allow them to move. Feet are parallel, about four to eight inches apart (wider if your thighs touch). Hips continually move very high toward the ceiling. Be sure you isolate your hamstring stretch before proceeding.

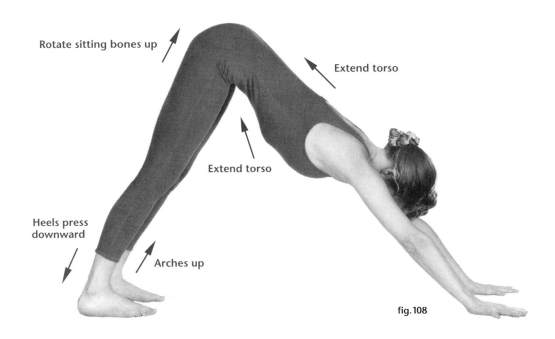

Rotate sitting bones up

Extend torso

Extend torso

Heels press downward

Arches up

fig. 108

Attitude Adjustment

▶ ***Aggressive***

Begin with the props. It is smarter to use them than prematurely going to the floor and increasing your potential for frustration or injury. Always keep your knees bent and your heels high to avoid any discomfort or pain in your knees or back. Don't stay too long in Down Dog (or any exercise) until you feel comfortable. Then slowly build your endurance by staying longer.

▶ ***Moderate & Easygoing***

Pay attention to the details and begin to lengthen the time you stay in the Dog pose. Work on lengthening your spine by rotating your hips up high. If you feel any pain or discomfort behind your knees, bend your knees a little more, or lift your heels a little higher, or both.

FINE-TUNING

hands *— Keep all four points of your hands actively pressing down.*

biceps and elbows *— Your biceps should rotate upward while your inner elbows should rotate slightly inward. Use the "headlight" image as seen in Figure 104 (page 96).*

head and shoulders *— Keep shoulders widening as in Figure 98 (page 94), not scrunching up as in Figure 99.*

hips and pelvis *— Always keep sitting bones lifting upward to engage hamstrings.*

knees *— Always keep knees slightly to deeply bent, depending on hamstring tightness.*

feet *— Press down evenly both inner and outer toe mounts. Even though your heels may be off the floor, press the inner and outer heels downward as well but keep arches lifting up.*

If you find that you cannot control your hands or feet, that they are sliding out away from you, place your hands against a wall, stretching your thumb away from your index finger and placing the "V" as close to the wall as possible. My favorite is to place both hands and feet on a thin, nonslip sticky mat (see Resources in Appendix VI), which I also use for the Standing postures, which follow.

Lunge (Again)

When you start doing your Sun Salutation sequence, you'll be coming back into a Lunge from the Downward Facing Dog pose by bringing your left foot forward to line up with your hands again. *This movement can be tricky and deserves some practice on its own.*

► **Tight to Moderate**

If your body is a little stiff, or if you're a beginner, it may be difficult for you to bring your left foot smoothly all the way forward into the Lunge. Instead, from Downward Facing Dog, just come down to your hands and knees. Then bring your left foot all the way forward so that it ends up between your hands. Pick your foot up with your left hand if you need to, assisting it all the way forward [Fig.109]. Do it this way as long as necessary, making a smoother transition as you become more skilled. You will soon find that as you become more flexible (and stronger), you'll be able to bring your left foot forward directly from the Downward Facing Dog in a smooth, flowing movement. Challenge yourself by testing it out after a week or two of practice.

► **Flexible**

If you're fairly flexible, from Downward Facing Dog you can simply rise up high on your toes and bring your left foot forward. Your right knee comes down to the floor and away from you as you move into the Lunge stretch. Make sure your left knee ends up directly over your left ankle.

FINE-TUNING

One final note about moving from Lunge to Down Dog to Lunge: **breathe.** *You will find that it is easier to make the transition while you are exhaling than if you hold your breath or even while you are inhaling.*

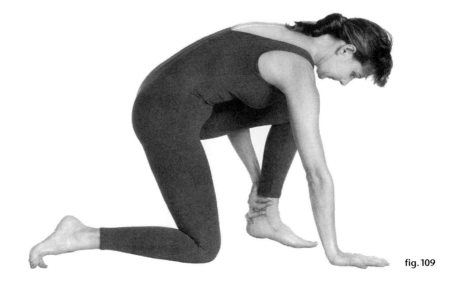

fig. 109

Alternate Hamstring Stretch from the Lunge

The Hamstring Stretch from the Lunge is another optional exercise, not usually part of the Sun Salutation sequence. It's a great way, however, to stretch your legs and is especially appropriate for Tight to Moderate body types. And it's still another good way to isolate a hamstrings stretch — try it if you've been having trouble feeling that. You can do it at any point when you're in a Lunge position.

Start from your Lunge position, one foot forward, one foot back, hands on the floor parallel with toes (you may need to stay up on your fingertips).

Variation #1: Inhale and press your torso to your forward thigh. As you exhale, slowly bring your back knee off the floor and begin to straighten it, very gradually. Keep your torso glued to your forward thigh [Figs.110, Tight, and 111, Moderate to Flexible]. Now slowly lengthen your forward leg, still keeping your torso in place. At this point, you'll start to feel an isolated stretch in your forward hamstrings. Don't straighten either leg all the way unless you can do so completely without discomfort or pain and still keep your torso in contact with your thigh. (Even I can't fully lengthen the forward leg all the way.) Hold the stretch, breathing evenly for two to eight breaths, then come back down to the Lunge position. Switch legs. Do each leg three to six times, breathing deeply on the stretch.

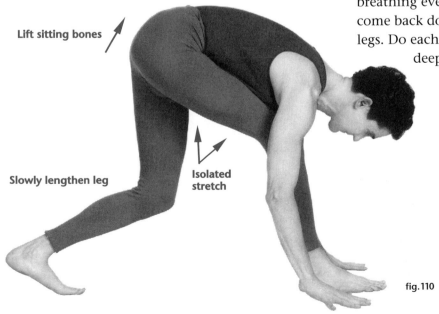

Lift sitting bones

Slowly lengthen leg

Isolated stretch

fig.110

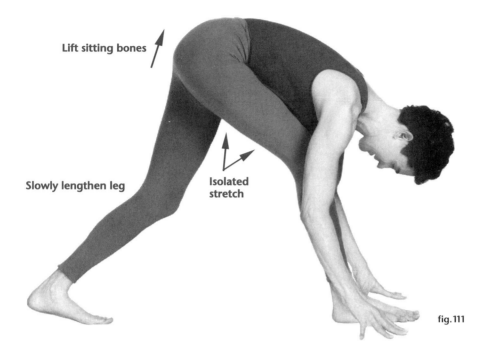

Lift sitting bones

Slowly lengthen leg

Isolated stretch

fig.111

Variation #2: Inhale. As you exhale, take your buttocks back toward your rear heel, slowly straightening your forward leg, dorsiflexing the foot [Fig.112]. Leave your back knee on the floor and your ribs resting on your front thigh. Keep your hands in place next to your forward foot (you'll probably have to come up on your fingertips). Keep moving your hips back gently until you feel a stretch in your forward hamstring. Stop at that point and breathe evenly. Hold the stretch for two to eight deep, even breaths, then come back to the Lunge position. Switch legs. Do each leg three to six times breathing deeply on the stretch.

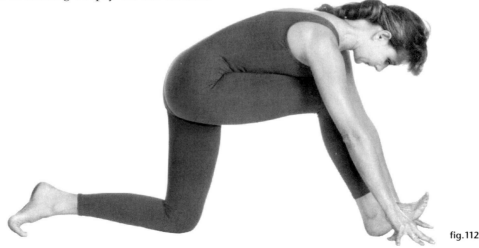

fig.112

Completing the Sun Salutation

To complete the Sun Salutation from the Lunge simply move your rear foot parallel with your forward foot and rest for a moment with your torso on your folded legs [Figs. 113A, 114A, 115A]. Then extend your torso into the Forward Bend appropriate for your body type [Figs. 113B, 114B, 115B]. Place your hands on your hips and be sure that you have isolated the stretch in your hamstrings before you go on (you might need to lift your torso a little higher or bend your knees a little bit more to isolate your hamstring stretch). Then, keeping your knees slightly bent, gently tuck your tailbone down and extend your arms out sideways while you begin rotating up (remember to rotate from your hips, not your shoulders). As you are standing up, take your arms over your head into the Arm Flap appropriate for your body type [Figs. 113C, 114C, 115C]. Adjust your shoulders downward to release any tension from your neck before you complete the routine by extending the arms, again sideways, back to your sides, ending up in the Mountain pose [Figs. 113D, 114D, 115D].

Tight Sequence

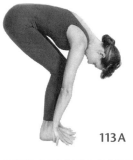

113A

Moderate Sequence

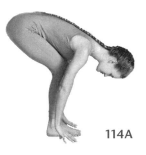

114A

Flexible Sequence

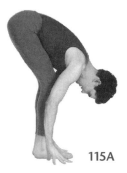

115A

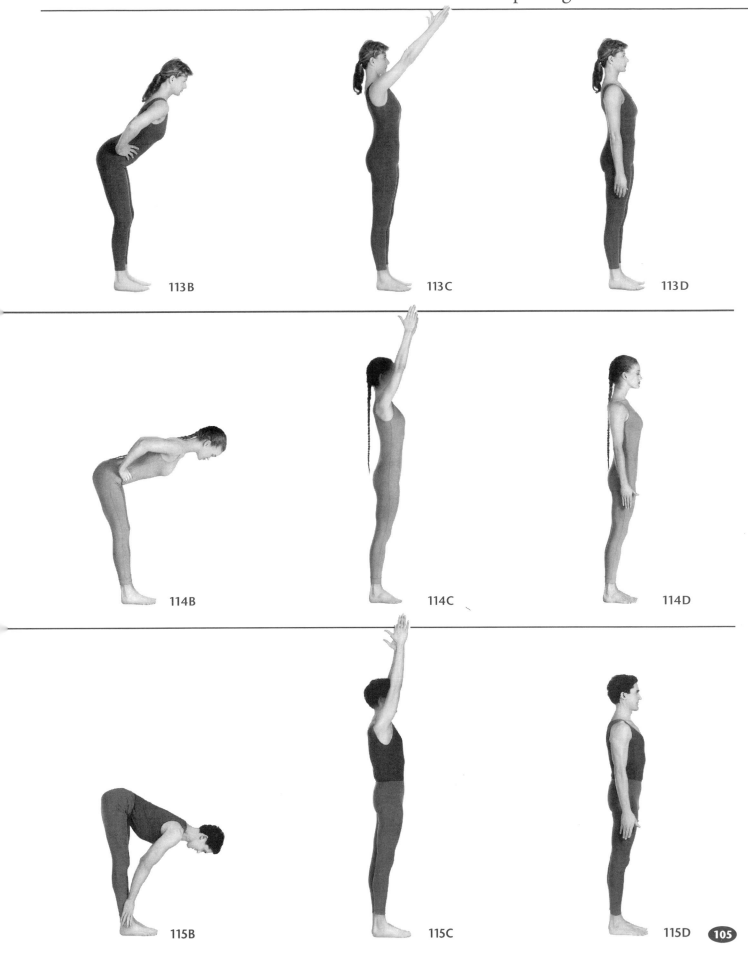

113B

113C

113D

114B

114C

114D

115B

115C

115D

FINE-TUNING

*When you put the entire sequence together and begin doing repetitive Sun Salutations, you'll need to keep track of which leg you are taking back and which leg you are bringing forward. You always start with your left foot; meaning that, for the first Lunge, you'll take your **left foot back and keep your right foot forward**, knee over ankle. After you go through the Plank, the Pose of the Child, the Cobra, and the Downward Facing Dog, you then bring your **left foot forward**, so that your left knee will be over its ankle and your **right foot and leg will be back** in the Lunge pose. You will then continue on into the standing Forward Bend, Arm Flap, and Mountain poses.*

*When you do your second Sun Salutation, you will take your **right foot back**, into Lunge, and your **left will be forward**. Continue on. Then after the Downward Facing Dog, you will bring your **right foot forward leaving your left foot and leg back**.*

*In other words, all **odd-numbered** repetitions begin with the **left foot back**, then bring the left foot forward. During all **even-numbered** repetitions you take your **right foot back**, then bring it forward.*

Putting It All Together

The final step is to put all of the separate exercises together, making a complete Sun Salutation.

First, *practice each posture slowly three or four times, getting used to each one on its own.*

Second, *practice the above sequences going from one pose to the next, and back again, so you know how it all feels.*

Third, *put all the poses together in order as described on pages 114–115.*

Remember These Principles:

1. Do not bounce in any of the postures or stretches (remember that less will always get you more).

2. Do not push or pull into discomfort or pain (remember Principle #2: Pain is a message that something is wrong and needs to be changed).

3. Keep your hands active.

4. Keep your arms and legs extended where appropriate.

5. Lengthen your spine, including your neck (Deer Ears) in all poses (ExTension releases tension).

6. Never try anything that hurts, especially in or behind your knees, into your sitting bones, lower back, or neck.

7. From Down Dog to Lunge, pick up your feet with your hands any time it's necessary.

Get into the practice of doing the complete Sun Salutation a minimum of two to four times on each side along with the rest of this program. Every day, four to six days a week. Follow the sequence for your body type. Every day, start very slowly. Take your time. Once you isolate the sensations — the actions, stretches, and flexes — in the appropriate body parts, you may go as quickly as you like doing as many repetitions as you wish.

The Sun Salutation Routine

One final thought about breathing before we begin: You will notice from the instructions on pages 114–115, each Sun Salutation movement has a specific inhalation or exhalation associated with it. Most beginners have difficulty coordinating the breathing with specific Sun Salutation movements. Don't be concerned right now about mastering the specific inhalations or exhalations, but always remember to breathe deeply and smoothly throughout all the routines.

I recommend that you mark these pages and refer to them often until you feel that you can "breathe with the movements."

A written description of the entire Sun Salutation follows on pages 114–115.

Here we go...

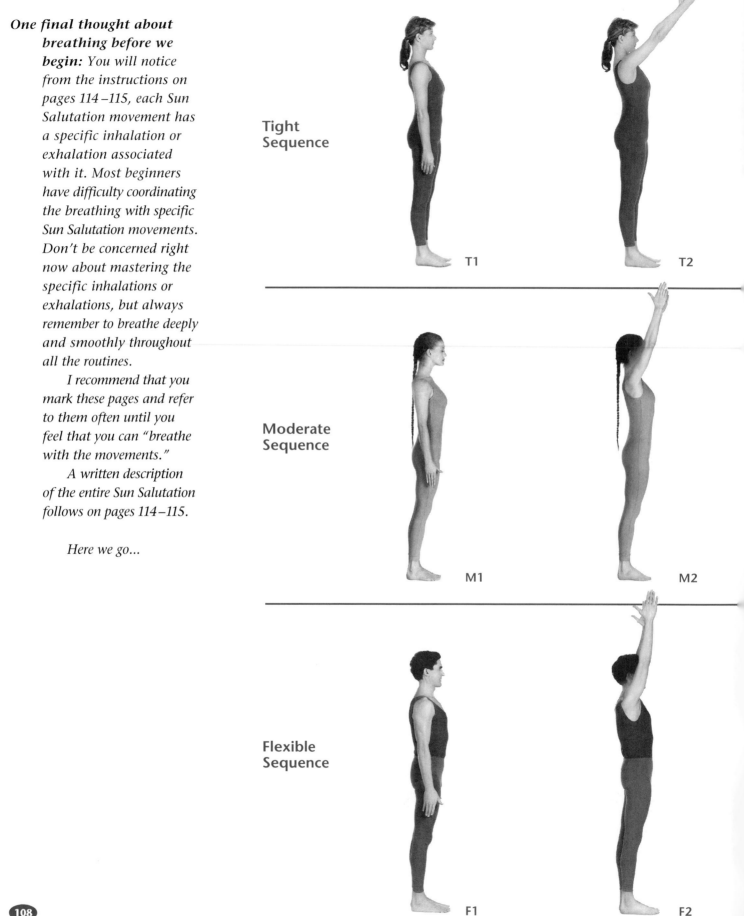

Tight Sequence

T1   T2

Moderate Sequence

M1   M2

Flexible Sequence

F1   F2

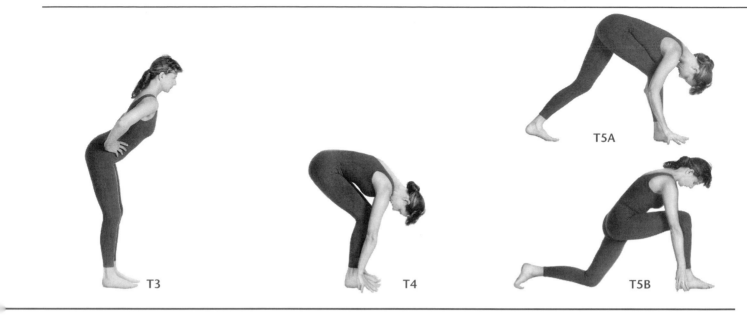

T3

T4

T5A

T5B

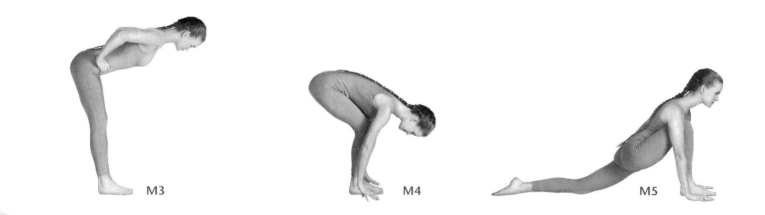

M3

M4

M5

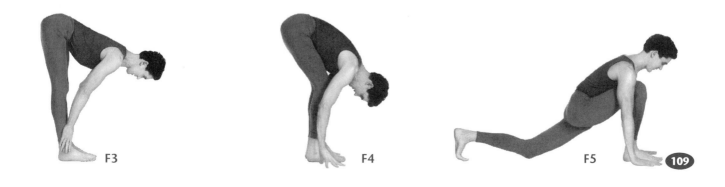

F3

F4

F5

**Tight
Sequence**

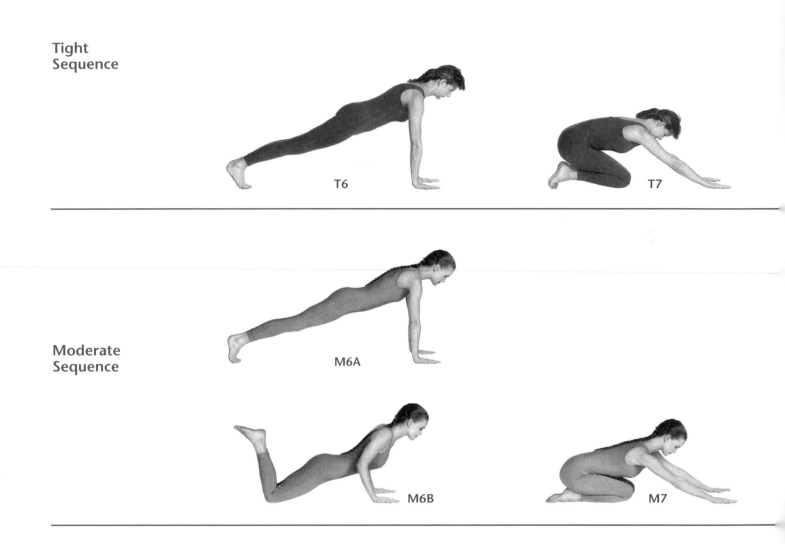

T6

T7

**Moderate
Sequence**

M6A

M6B

M7

**Flexible
Sequence**

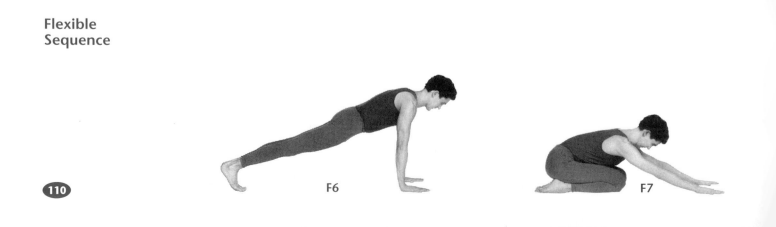

F6

F7

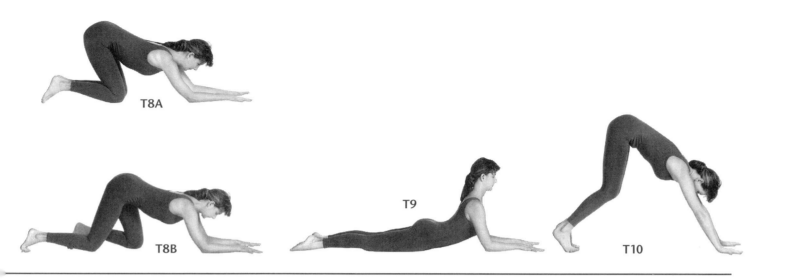

T8A

T8B

T9

T10

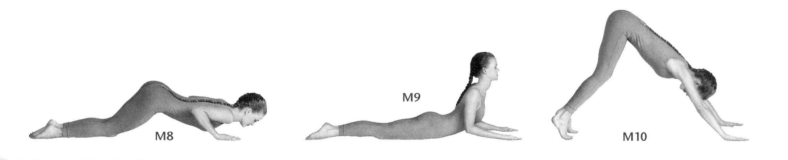

M8

M9

M10

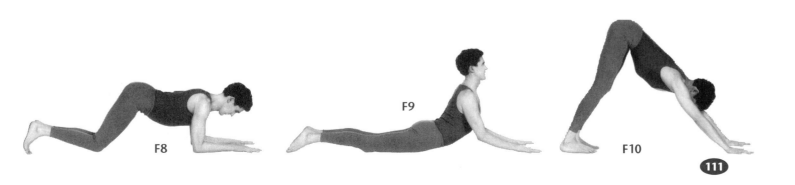

F8

F9

F10

**Tight
Sequence**

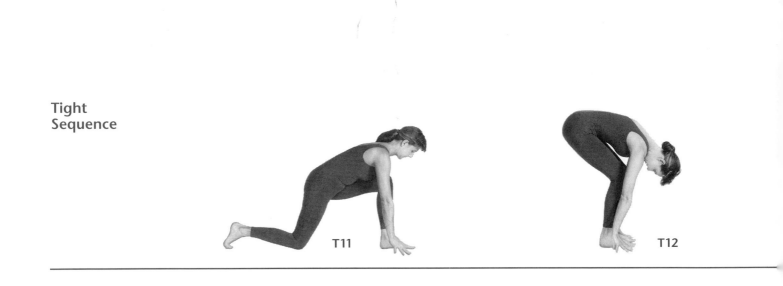

T11

T12

**Moderate
Sequence**

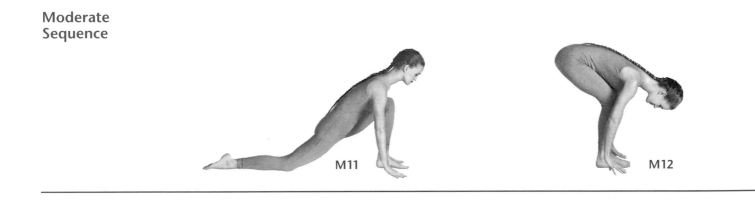

M11

M12

**Flexible
Sequence**

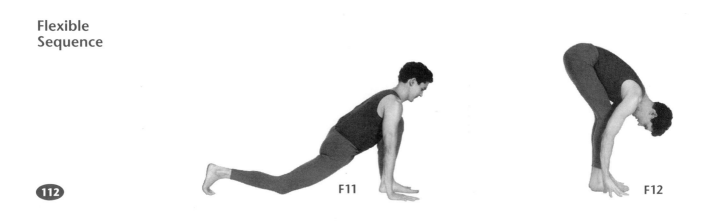

F11

F12

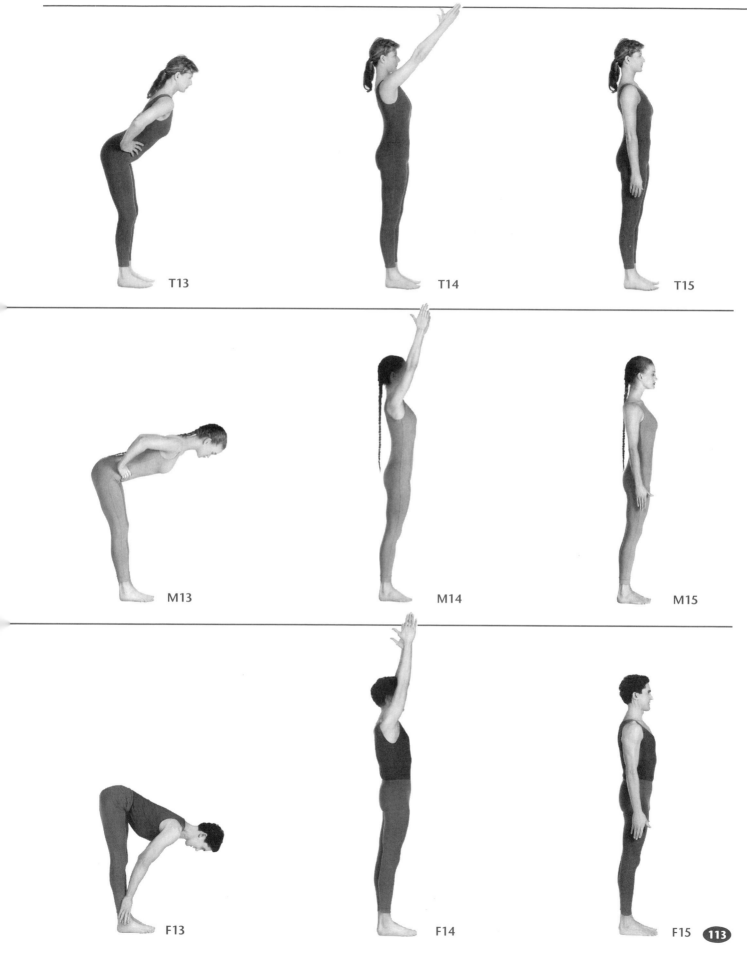

T13　　　　　T14　　　　　T15

M13　　　　　M14　　　　　M15

F13　　　　　F14　　　　　F15

1. ***Stand in Mountain pose*** [Figs. T1, M1, F1]: Hands at your sides with deep and easy breathing. "Grow taller" from your feet up through your neck and head.

2. ***Arm Flap*** [Figs. T2, M2, F2]: Activate your hands by stretching your palms — the thumb away from the fingers. Slowly inhale while extending your arms sideways up and over your head. Relax your neck by keeping your shoulders down and wide.

3. ***Forward Bend*** [Figs. T3, M3, F3]: Exhale keeping your arms and hands active while you bring your hands to your hips. Remember to bend your knees and rotate your torso from your hips. Lift up on your sitting bones and feel your spine growing longer. Feel the stretching action in your hamstrings. If you like, you can hold for two to four long, deep, and easy breaths while exploring the stretches.

4. ***Prepare for the Lunge (fold over)*** [Figs. T4, M4, F4]: Slowly begin inhaling while you move, bending your knees and placing your fingertips on either side of your feet, belly on thighs, fingertips in line and parallel with toes, and continue directly to…

5. ***Lunge*** [Figs. T5, M5, F5]: During the same inhalation, place your left knee on the floor behind you. The right knee stays directly over the right heel. Keeping your left knee on the floor, slide it back until you feel an action in your hips, groins, or thigh. If you like, you can hold for two to four long deep and easy breaths.
    Lunge Options — Right hamstring stretches, Variations 1 and 2 shown in Tight Sun Salutation sequences [Figs. T5A and T5B] only. Hold for two to four long breaths while exploring the stretches.

6. ***Plank*** [Figs. T6, M6, F6]: Exhale, keep your hands in place, and put your left foot back next to your right foot, stretching through your elbows and keeping your body straight as a board.
    Plank variation — shown in Moderate Sun Salutation sequence [Fig. M6B] only: Continuing to exhale, place your knees on the floor (sliding them back just far enough so that your arms remain perpendicular to the floor). Then bend your knees so that your feet are toward the ceiling. Keeping your hands in place directly under your shoulders, bend your elbows and inhale as you lower your torso toward the floor (go down only as far as you can comfortably come up). Exhale as you are pushing up. Repeat two to ten times.

7. ***Pose of the Child*** [Figs. T7, M7, F7]: From Plank, take a deep, long, slow, inhalation while you are moving into the Pose of the Child. Keep your hands in place and sit on or close to your heels with arms extended, shoulder width apart (scoot knees closer to or farther from hands as necessary). Pull the floor toward you without moving your hands. Keep your head up, spine and neck long (Deer Ears). Hold for two to four breaths while pulling your arms and extending your spine during each exhalation. Then begin exhaling while you make the transition to the Cobra pose.

8. **_Transition to Cobra_** [Figs. T8A and B, M8, F8]: Easy one-leg-at-a-time transition to Cobra is shown in Tight Sun Salutation sequence Figures T8A and B only. Continue to exhale, sliding your feet away from you (one at a time if necessary), toes extended.

9. **_Cobra_** [Figs. T9, M9, F9]: Inhale slowly, keeping your hands in place, and pull the floor toward you to activate your triceps, but keep your elbows bent and no wider than your shoulders. Lift your chest and pull your spine and belly long. If you like, you can hold for two to four deep breaths (finish on an inhalation), then come to hands and knees.

10. **_Downward Facing Dog_** [Figs. T10, M10, F10]: Exhale while you come onto your hands and knees and lift your hips up into Dog pose. Walk your feet toward your hands three to six inches and isolate the stretch in the hamstrings by lifting up on the sitting bones (don't forget to keep knees bent). Keep your hands secure to the floor, stretch your elbows and lift your chest. Don't let your head drop; line it up with your arms. As an option, you can hold the Dog pose for four to ten breaths, then come back to your hands and knees.

11. **_Lunge_** [Figs. T11, M11, F11]: Inhale, step your left foot forward, toes in line with fingertips, left knee directly over its ankle. Slide your right knee back on the floor until you feel an action in your hips, groin, or thigh.
    Lunge Option — Left hamstring stretching, not shown, but same as #5 with left leg forward. Hold for two to four long, deep, and easy breaths.

12. **_Preparation for Forward Bend (fold over)_** [Figs. T12, M12, F12]: Begin exhalation. Step your right foot forward in line with your left, knees bent, hands on the floor, belly on thighs and continue directly to...

13. **_Forward Bend_** [Figs. T13, M13, F13]: During the same exhalation, place your hands on your hips as you bring your torso up into your forward bend. Lift your sitting bones; feel your hamstrings stretch. Move on, or hold for two to four long, deep and easy breaths while exploring the stretches.

14. **_Arm Flap_** [Figs. T14, M14, F14]: Inhale while bringing your arms sideways up overhead, hands active.

15. **_Mountain pose_** [Figs. T15, M15, F15]: Exhale and lower your active arms and hands sideways to your body. Stand quietly and breathe deeply.

Repeat, starting with your right foot back. Do as many complete sequences as you want. Then do the standing and floor exercises that follow and conclude with relaxation.

The Sun Salutation Routine

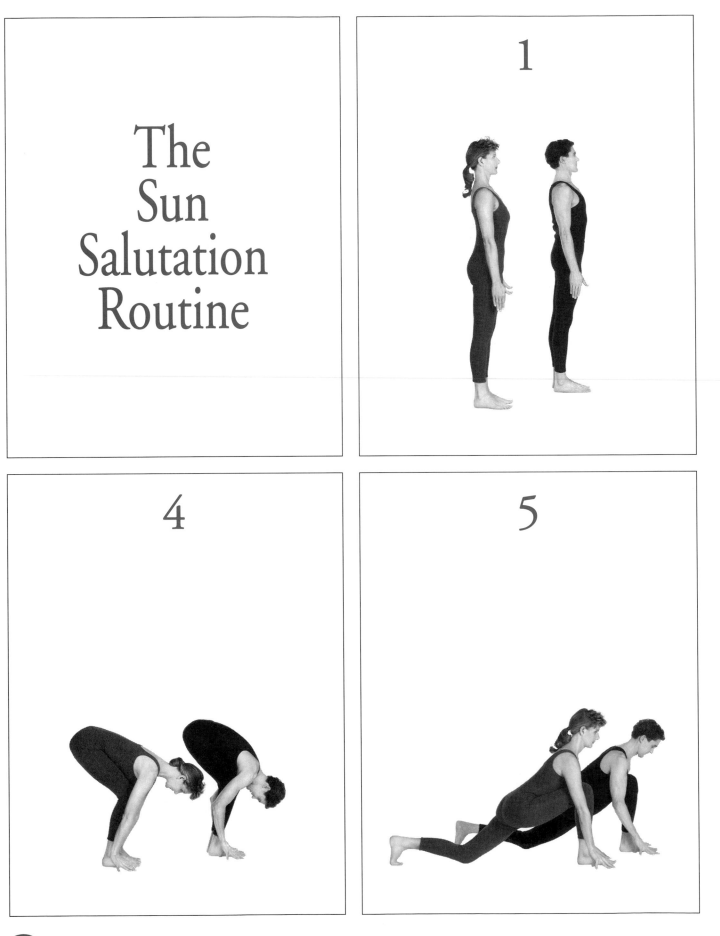

1

4

5

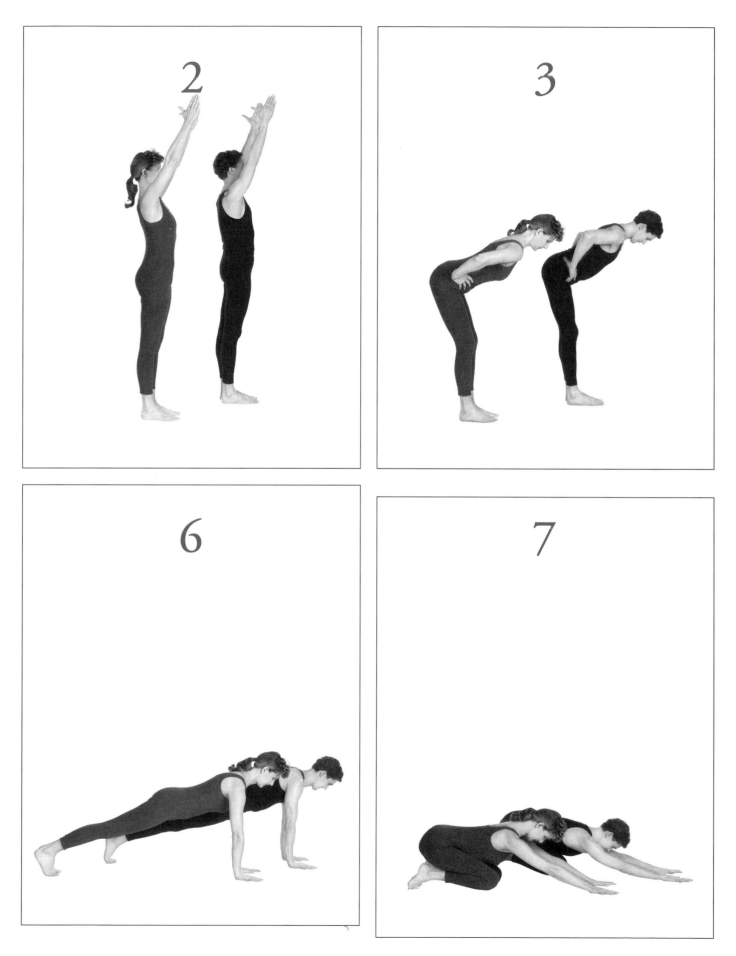

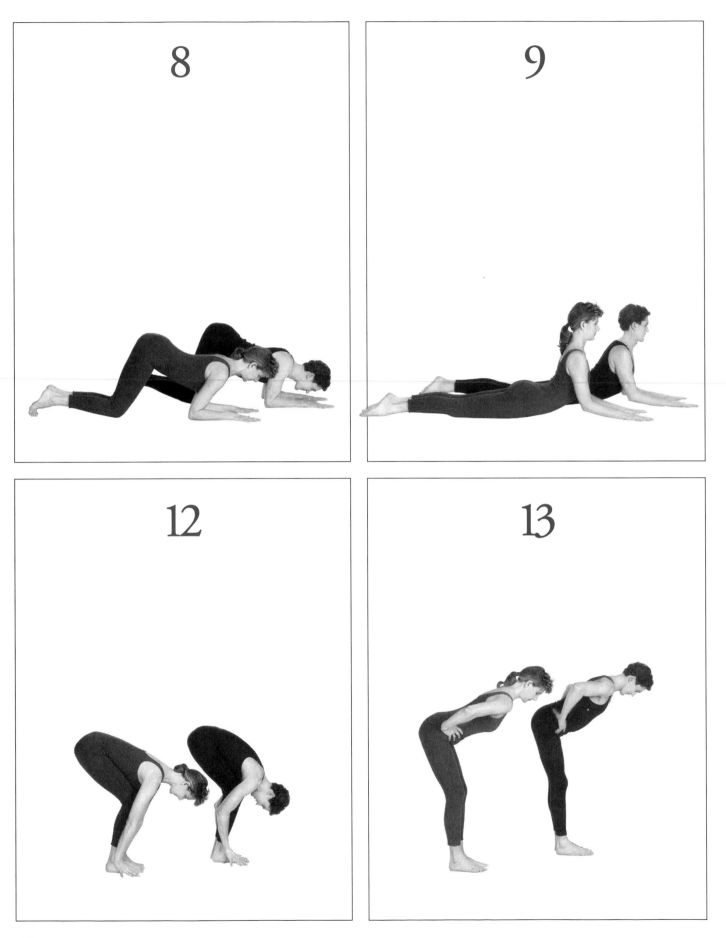

8

9

12

13

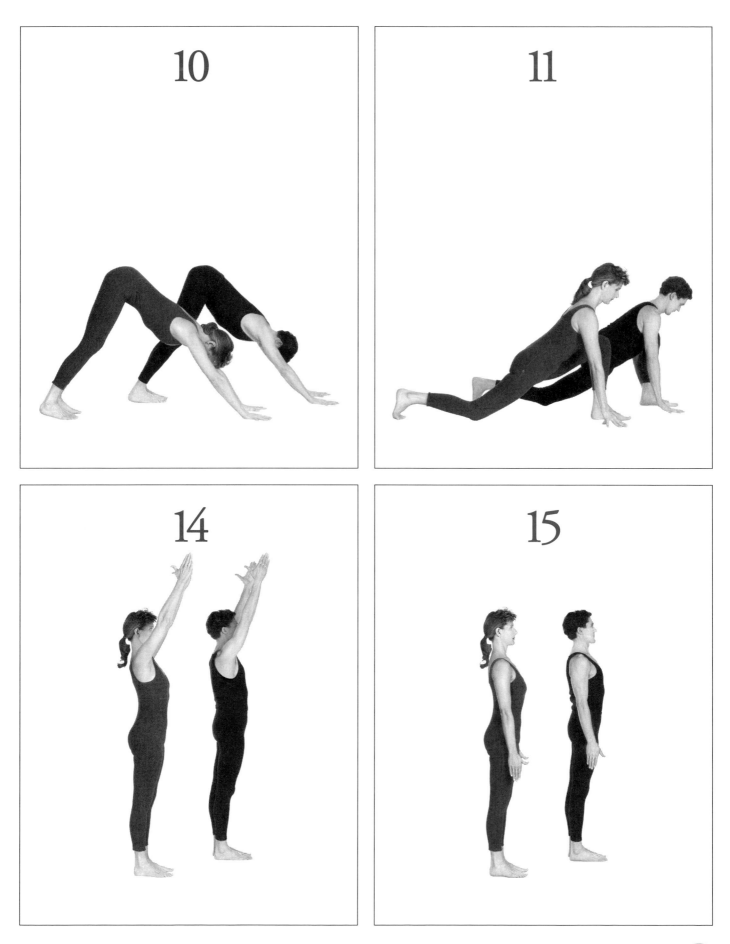

Practice Tip: Notes on an Extended Practice

Done just 20 minutes a day, four to six days a week, the entire program, including Sun Salutations, will contribute to an overall feeling of well-being and fitness. If you wish, you can use Sun Salutations to build cardiovascular fitness. You can even put on some music that you like.

For instance, when I am moving slowly, I like to listen to classical music. When I set a faster pace I like to play more contemporary, faster music. As you get better at the Sun Salutations, you'll begin to work up a sweat with repeated sequences. For cardiovascular enhancement, practice 20 to 25 minutes without stopping. An accomplished practitioner — of any flexibility — can do as many as 100 Sun Salutations in 20 to 25 minutes. But do not push yourself past what you can do at any given stage. Take your time, adhere to the details, and build up your repetitions. Have fun with it and make them flow. After you have completed your Sun Salutations, whether it be four to a hundred, conclude with the remainder of the program.

But on any given day, if you're doing just Sun Salutations and not going on to the entire program, be sure to go to page 160 for a few minutes of relaxation practice.

The three standing postures you're about to learn are powerful strengtheners for your entire body, but they will especially firm up, strengthen, and tone your legs. Done faithfully and correctly, they can also restore mobility and flexibility to Tight legs and hips and help build cardiovascular endurance (and if held after repetitive Sun Salutations, a vigorous sweat). They will refresh and energize you.

Do these exercises barefoot, on a hard, nonslippery surface, with room to stretch out your arms and legs. You may need to clear space against a wall so you can use it for balance and to help keep your back foot from slipping as you are learning the postures. (If your feet slide during standing postures, you won't feel comfortable enough to hold them long enough to do any good.) You can also stand on a thin, nonslip sticky mat (see Resources in Appendix VI) placed in the middle of the room. Sticky mats are excellent for holding your hands in the Downward Facing Dog pose as well. You'll notice a few sticky mats in the following photographs (our working surface wasn't slippery, but we wanted occasionally to show the postures on mats).

Before You Start

Because these are standing exercises, it's extremely important to review your basic standing position, the Mountain pose. Make sure that your feet are reasonably parallel, two to three inches apart (more if your knees touch), and that you feel equal weight on all four points of each foot: the inner heel, outer heel, inner ball mount, and outer ball mount. Then draw up your arches while lengthening your toes. Continue extending up through your kneecaps and up into your torso.

Pull your spine long, ears away from your shoulders (Deer Ears), and turn your head a couple of times to release any tension in your neck. Check that your shoulders are relaxed and down. Make a mental run-through of your posture before and during the standing exercises.

As you look at the photographs, you will notice that our models are turning to the right side as you are looking at them. All our instructions will have you starting the exercises by *going to the right* so that you can *mirror* the examples. Then do the same exercise on the left side. As you work on both sides, you may notice that you are more flexible or that you feel more or less discomfort on one side or the other. This is completely normal.

Foot positioning is crucial to holding these postures safely and effectively. The best surface for standing postures is a wood floor because it is so easy to align the feet with the lines of the floorboards and because wood, a natural substance, is more comfortable to stand on than concrete, tile, or linoleum. If possible, use a sticky mat on very hard or slippery surfaces. The worst surface for standing postures is soft, thick piled carpet because it is so hard to activate the feet and lift through the spine.

fig.116

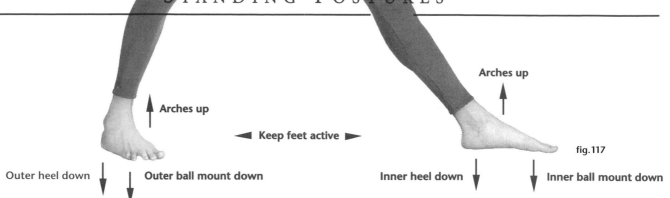

Arches up

Arches up

↑ Keep feet active ▶

Outer heel down   ↓ Outer ball mount down   Inner heel down ↓   ↓ Inner ball mount down

fig. 117

For all three of the standing poses, you will step your feet wide apart. Let's test this now. Step your feet about three to three and a half feet apart and keep them parallel. As you do this, keep the integrity of your Mountain pose — evenly distributed weight, feet parallel to start, long, lifted spine, relaxed shoulders and neck [Fig. 116 (page 121), on sticky mat].

From your feet-parallel position, you will begin by turning your right foot (I'll always have you start with your right foot) a full 90 degrees to the right. Your rear, or left, foot will turn inward about about half that distance, toes toward the inside. To rotate your front foot, just leave your heel where it is, pick your toes up, pivot on your heel, and put your toes down. Now press down and activate your feet (arches lift while the inner and outer heels and the inner and outer ball mounts press down) [Fig. 117] Test out this position now, and keep the heel of your right foot lined up with the heel of your left.

If this is at all uncomfortable or you are having difficulty with your balance, move your right foot two to three inches more to the side, so that if you were to draw a line from your right heel toward your back foot, that line would pass just behind your left heel by two to three inches.

Again, foot placement is critical. If your feet are not firmly and correctly placed on the floor — the right foot turned out a full 90 degrees with the center of your right knee directly in line with the center of your right foot and the left foot slightly turned in — there is a possibility of straining your knees. This leads to irritation and contraction of soft tissue — which is exactly what we want to avoid with any of these exercises. Always remember that

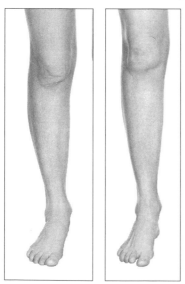

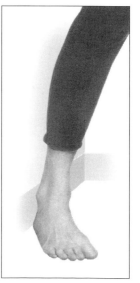

with the standing exercises — and all the exercises in ExTension — forcing or straining only works against you. On the other hand, to create beneficial change, you must be willing to challenge yourself intelligently (observing all the cautions), but you also must know when to back off to avoid pain and strain.

A fine point that will help you hold your standing postures is lifting your kneecaps. Activate your feet by lifting your arches up while pressing the inner ball mounts and inner heels of the feet down. Further activate your feet by extending your toes wide and onto the floor, then draw your knees up by contracting your quadriceps (your front thigh

fig. 118   fig. 119

fig. 120

muscles). Feel as if you are Tightening them upward [Fig. 118, sagging kneecaps, Fig. 119, lifted kneecaps]. This takes some practice — if you can't tell when you're doing it, place your hand on your kneecap and feel it move up when you contract your quadriceps. While you're doing the standing poses, keep your kneecaps drawn up, *but never locked or pushed back*. If you find your kneecaps locking or pushing back, not up, you'll need to bend your knees slightly. Then the kneecaps will come up.

For all of the standing poses, work in the middle of the room if you can, but if you feel at all unsure of your balance or strength, you may stand with your rear heel braced against the wall [Fig.120]. You'll still turn both feet as instructed above. The wall support simply helps keep you from falling over, sliding, or putting too much stress on untrained muscles (sliding feet usually means that you have not yet learned how to keep your feet active).

Let's do one more test before you start. Place your hands flat against your sides at your waist [Fig.121]. Notice that you feel the same on both sides. Now just drop your right shoulder and bend to the right a little. Can you feel the muscles bunch up on that side [Fig.122]? This bunching creates an imbalance in the muscles between the left and right sides of your spine. It disrupts the union and harmony that is created through yoga exercise. It puts tension in your lower back, setting off a possible chain reaction of contraction-pain-contraction that could lead to injury.

The way to avoid that possibility is always to lengthen the muscles along both sides of your spine equally, especially while moving into the Triangle pose and Extended Angle posture.

Ready? Here we go.

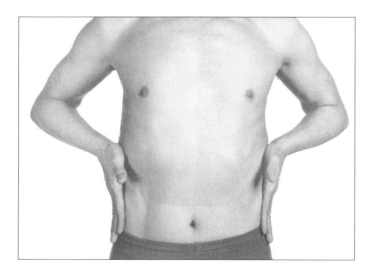

fig.121

fig.122

Triangle Pose

The purpose of the Triangle pose is to tone and firm your legs, especially your inner thighs.

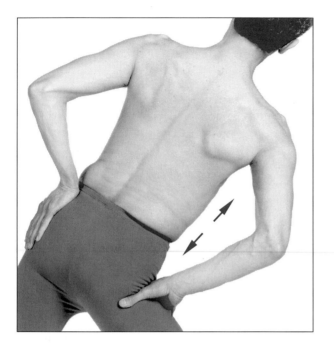

fig. 123

Begin by standing in the Mountain pose near the wall or in the middle of the room (remember, if you start in the middle of the room and experience any slipping, go to the wall or use a sticky mat).

Step your feet apart about three to three and a half feet wide, less wide if you have short legs, wider if you have long legs. Turn your right foot 90 degrees out toward the side and turn your left foot in about half that distance. If you are using the wall, stand sideways to it with your left heel braced against the baseboard.

Put your right hand on your right front hip (directly in the hip crease) and your left palm high on the back of your left hip, just above the buttock. Inhale, lift your spine long, and, instead of bending (dropping) over to your right side, lift your left hip up into your hand by simply cocking your pelvis up on that side [Fig.123]. Now, begin exhaling and simply move your hips back away from your right leg and away from your right hand (which is in the hip crease) until you feel a stretch in your right inner thigh. Your entire torso will rotate very slightly to the right as you do this.

Keep your *shoulders* parallel with the wall in front of you, but you *must* allow your left hip to come slightly forward; don't try to keep your hips parallel with the wall in front of you as you come into the pose. If you fail to move your left hip forward, a ridge on the top of the left hip socket will hit the head of the thigh bone and keep the pelvis from rotating along with the spine. That causes the lower back and sacral area to become stressed, ultimately causing irritation and pain.

Don't drop your ear down toward your right shoulder or lift your chin. Your spine should be long and straight and your head in a neutral position (remember your Deer Ears) [Fig.124].

Think about opening up your chest by taking your shoulders slightly back.

Both legs stay straight, knees lifting but not locked back. Feel a stretch, an action, in your right inner thigh. If you want to feel a deeper action, you can lift your left buttock higher. You don't need to bend your spine down into a curve at all.

Take your right hand and feel the right side of your waist and lower back. If you're doing this correctly, you won't feel any bunching; if you do, lift your torso and come back up all the way, rotating from your hips, not your shoulders. Then lengthen your spine, square your shoulders, left hip a little forward, and maintain that spinal length equally on the left and right sides as you rotate back down into the Triangle by lifting your left hip.

Hold the pose for about two to eight breaths, breathing evenly and keeping the weight evenly balanced between your right and left legs. If you start feeling pressure in your right (forward) leg or behind your left knee, press the outside of your left heel harder against the floor or wall. If you still feel discomfort behind your right knee, you may need to come up higher or bend the right knee just a fraction.

When you're ready to come up, bring both hands back to your waist, rotate your left hip back down, and lift up, moving your whole torso from your hips, and not just lifting your shoulders.

Switch the position of your feet and repeat the pose on the other side. Practice by doing the pose on one side, then the other, holding for two to eight breaths, until you've done two to four on each side.

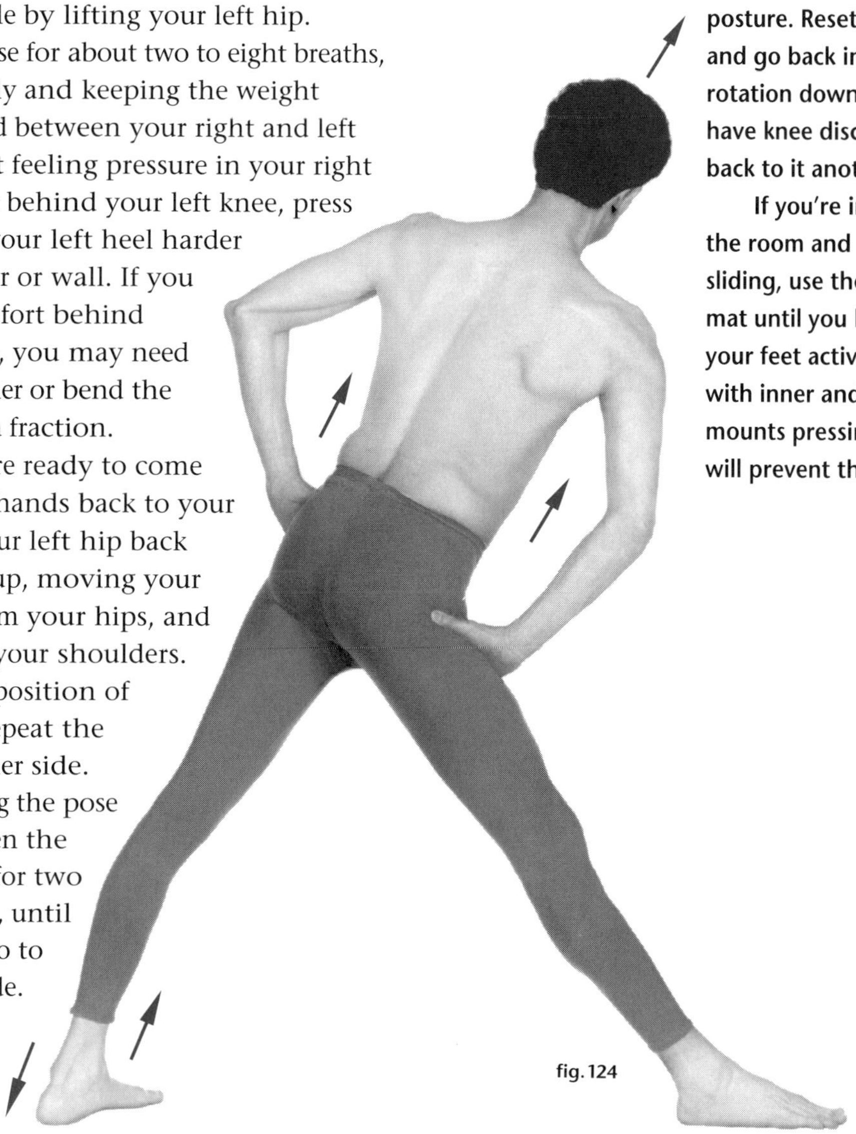

CAUTION

If you have knee problems, take extra care not to hyperextend (lock) your knees. If your front knee hurts in this or any other standing posture, slightly bend your front knee to take the pressure off, and use the wall or narrow your stance. If it still hurts, activate your feet and legs more. If you still experience pain, stop and come out of the posture. Reset your foundations and go back into it but with less rotation downward. If you still have knee discomfort, come back to it another day.

If you're in the middle of the room and feel your feet sliding, use the wall or a sticky mat until you learn how to keep your feet active (arches lifted with inner and outer ball mounts pressing down), which will prevent the sliding.

fig. 124

Triangle Pose

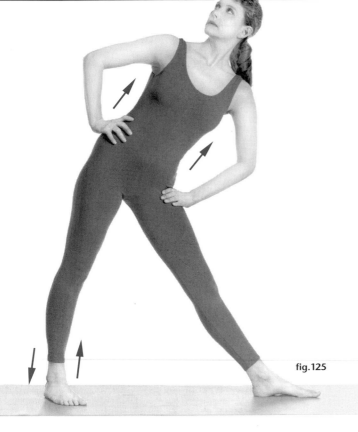

fig.125

► **Tight**

With your feet about three to three and a half feet apart, stand in the middle of the room [Fig.125] (using a sticky mat if you have one), or brace your left foot against the wall [Fig.126]. Be sure that the rear foot turns in, not out. Your right foot turns out 90 degrees, and its heel is aligned with the left heel. Or open your stance, if it feels better, by moving the right foot two to three inches farther to the right. For now, both hands remain on hips.

You will need to rotate your left hip forward and up only slightly before feeling a significant stretch in your inner right groin, or your thigh muscles, or both. Your head faces straight ahead as in Figure 126, or you may turn to look upward as in Figure 125. Regardless, be sure you maintain Deer Ears. Bend your right knee slightly if you have any back-of-knee pain [Fig.127].

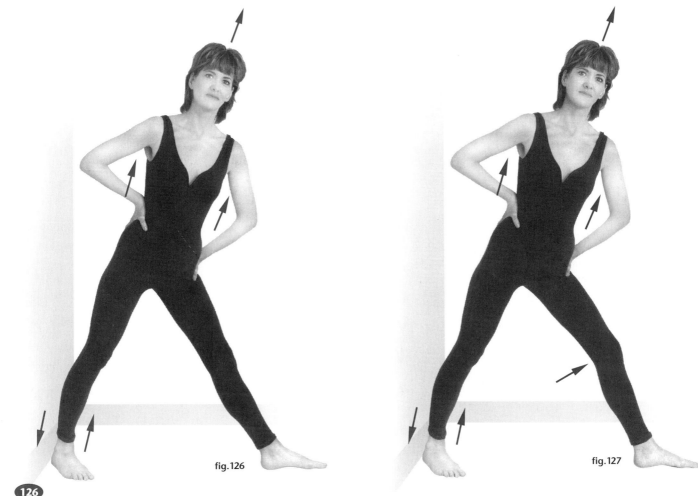

fig.126

fig.127

► **Moderate**

With your feet about three to three and a half feet apart, stand in the middle of the room (using a sticky mat if you have one). The heel of your right foot is aligned with the heel of your left foot. Your hands start out on your hips [Fig.128], but as you become more adept, your right hand can come down your leg somewhere between the knee and ankle (but don't press into the knee itself). Your left arm will then stretch up to the ceiling with an active hand and arm. Keep your shoulder blades moving wide. For a deeper stretch, take your legs just a little wider, rotating your left hip forward and a little higher. Your head can face straight ahead or can turn up to look at your overhead hand; either way, be sure to go keep your Deer Ears [Fig.129].

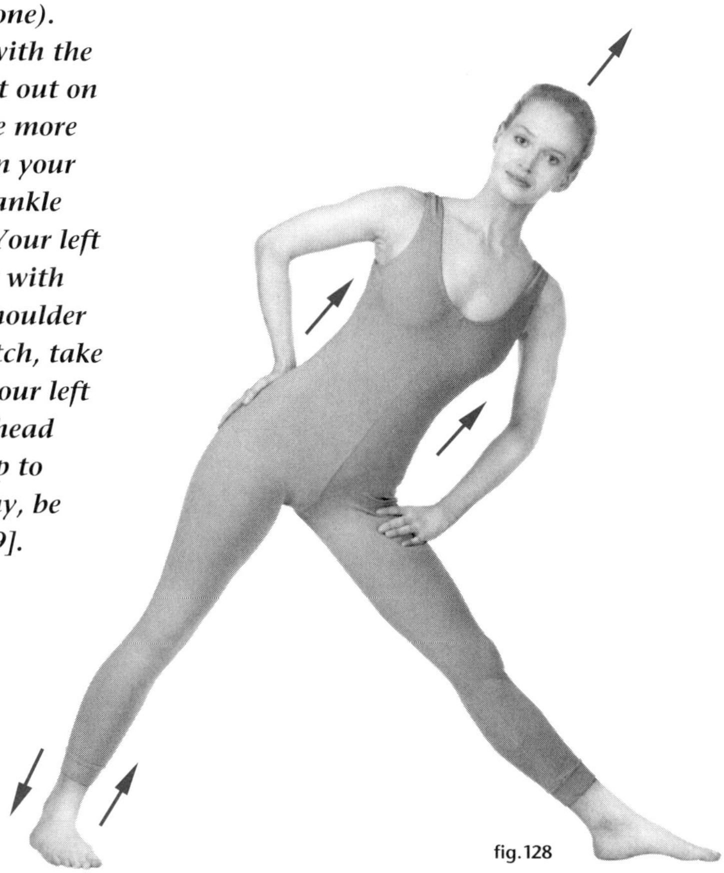

fig.128

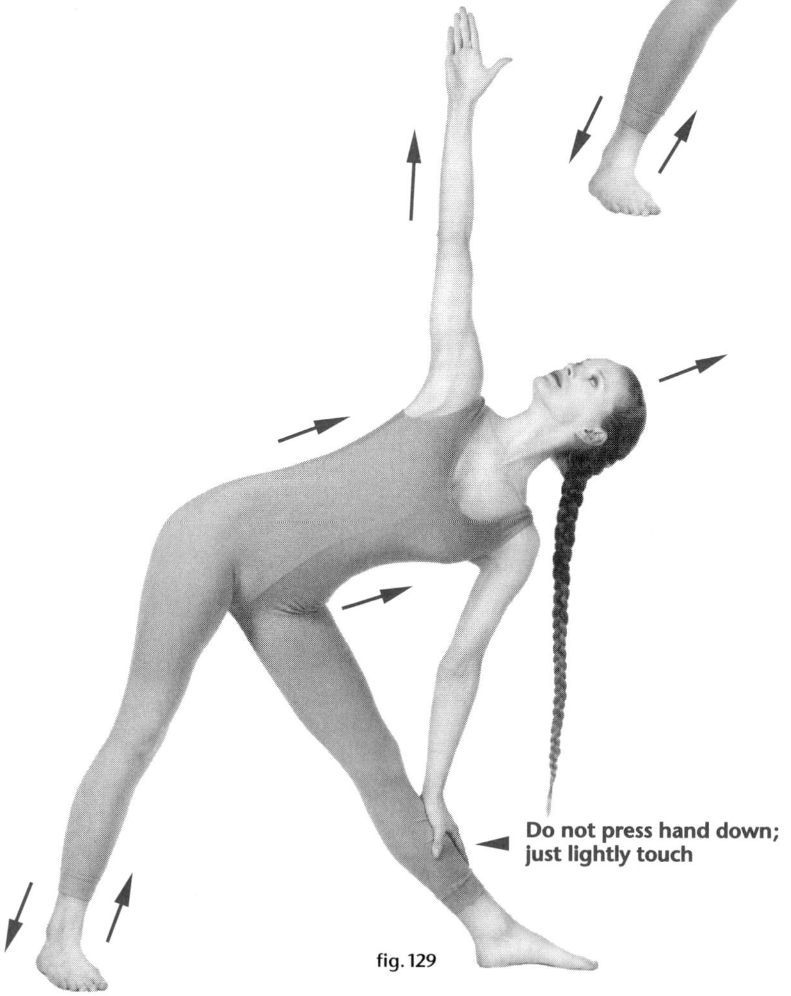

Do not press hand down; just lightly touch

fig.129

► **Flexible**

Begin by doing both Moderate examples above: first, hands on hips, then, left arm up and right arm on your leg. Then take your feet another few inches wider and rotate your left hip forward and up to allow right fingertips to move down toward ankle or floor, keeping both arms and hands equally active [Figs. 130 and 131]. Your head faces straight ahead or turns to look up at your left hand. Remember that the bottom side of your spine must stay long, not bent.

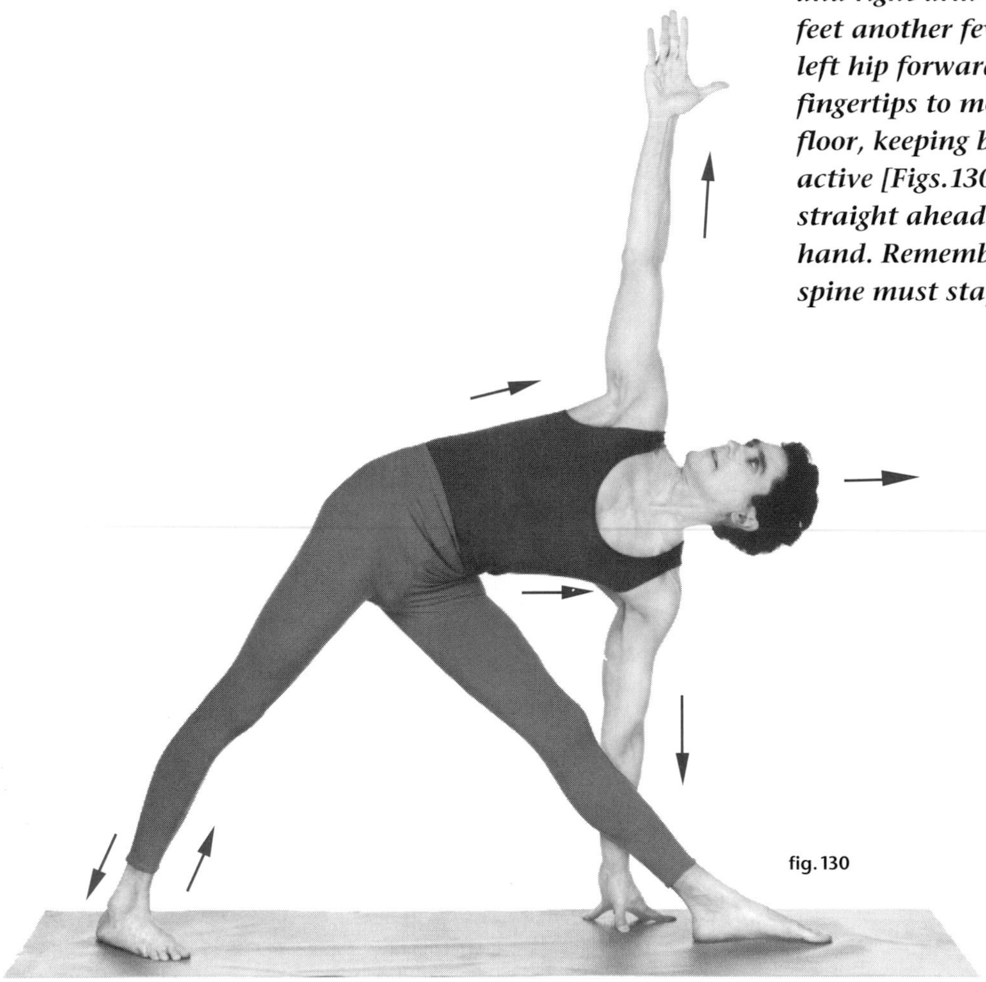

fig. 130

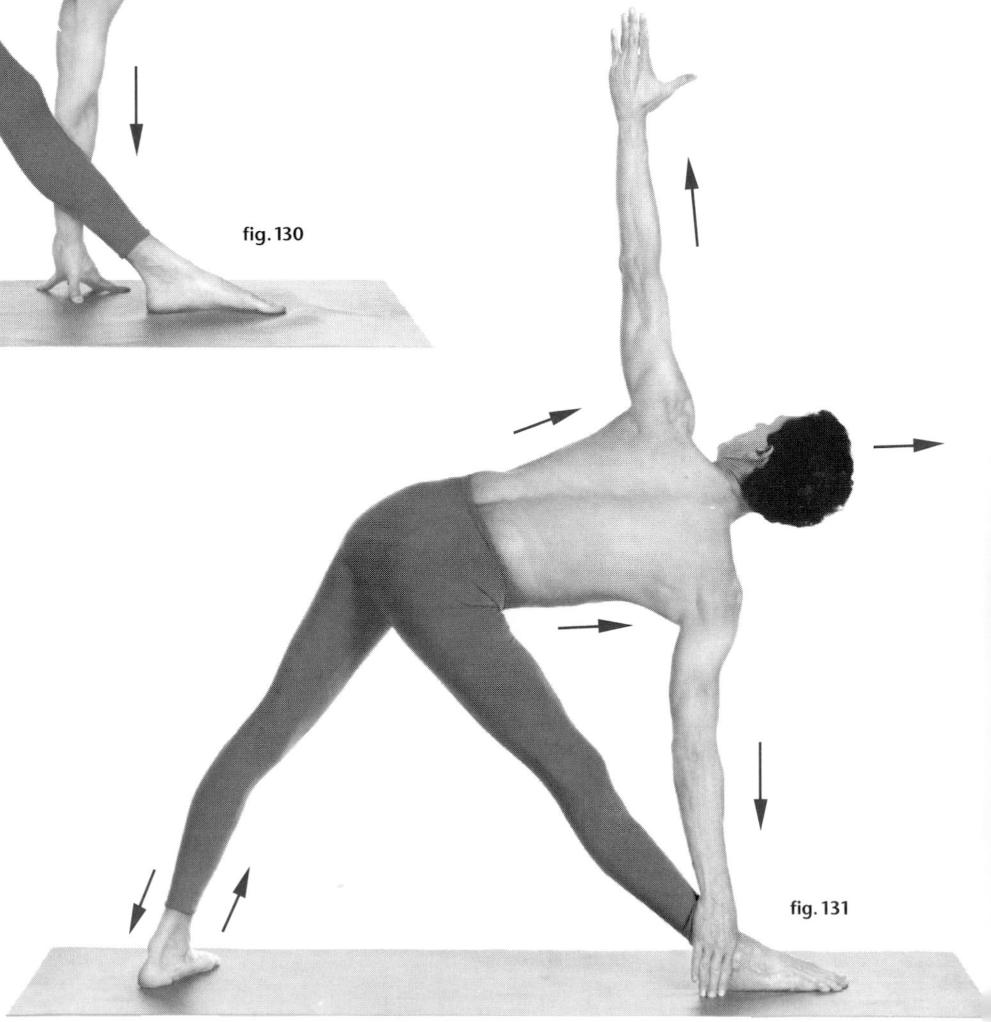

fig. 131

NOTE

If you were to compare this Triangle with the more traditional pose shown in Appendix II, you would notice how little effort and strain you experience in this position as compared with the other. This is another example in which less, done correctly, will always get you more.

Attitude Adjustment for Triangle and All of Your Standing Postures

► *Aggressive*

Start with the Tight adaptations, using the wall at first. Don't try to go too far. If you feel any discomfort, walk your feet narrower and follow the arrows upward to ease off on the pose. Allow your rear hip to rotate forward slightly to reduce the stress in your low back, pelvis, or groin. Once you get this, test it out in the middle of the room. Remember to relax your jaw and breathe deeply.

► *Moderate*

Start with the Tight adaptations. If you can do them without discomfort, especially in your knees or back, progress toward the Moderate examples right away. Depending on how you feel each day, challenge yourself by following the downward arrows and going lower or ease up on the pose by following the arrows upward.

► *Easygoing*

Start with the basic pose for a Tight body; if it comes easily to you, keep challenging yourself with more Flexible adaptations. Don't approach this lazily. Test your standing postures by going a little further — widen your stance and move in the direction of the downward arrows — each time you practice. But as always, never push into pain or discomfort.

WHAT YOU'LL FEEL

If you're doing this correctly, you will feel a definite stretch in the inner thigh of your forward leg, and both sides of your waist and spine will feel long and strong.

FINE-TUNING

Create a feeling that the arches of your feet are "sucking upward," as the four ball mounts of your feet actively and evenly press down. This should cause your inner thigh to stretch more, and you may even need to take your torso higher, out of the stretch.

You can also increase the action in the inner thigh of the forward leg by simply taking your feet a little bit wider or creating a little more lift in the rear pelvis. Always remember to rotate from the pelvis, not the spine.

The Warrior

The purpose of the Warrior pose is to tone and strengthen your arms and thighs and stretch your groin. Holding the pose also challenges the strength and endurance of your entire body.

If you were using the wall in the Triangle pose, you will probably start out by bracing your rear foot against it for the Warrior. If not, stay in the middle of the room, but if your feet start to slide, use the wall or a sticky mat.

From the Mountain pose, press your hands down on your hips and walk both feet equally apart, anywhere from four to four and a half feet wide (narrower for shorter legs, wider for longer legs). This will be wider than in the Triangle pose. Start with your feet parallel, then turn your right foot out 90 degrees and turn your left foot inward half that amount (about 30 to 45 degrees). All of the foot details you learned in the Triangle pose apply here as well.

Keeping your torso perpendicular to the floor, take a

◄ **Active feet** ►   fig. 132

◄ **Active feet** ►   fig.133

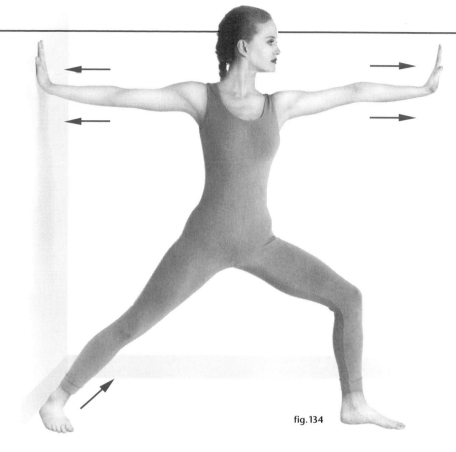

fig.134

long, deep inhalation and as you let it out, slowly bend your right knee until it's directly above your ankle [Fig.132]. If you're flexible it will come close to forming a 90-degree angle. If you are Tight you won't come down nearly as far (and that's okay). Keep your weight evenly distributed between *both* feet, and particularly focus your attention on the outside edge of your left foot by pressing it into the floor. Regardless of how wide you are, you should be able to look down and see that your right knee is just over your right ankle. If you can easily bend your knee beyond your ankle, you need to widen your stance. If you can't bring your knee over your ankle, you need to narrow your stance.

Establish a steady pose with your hips almost square — but, as in the Triangle, your left hip must come slightly forward to make the pose more comfortable in your right groin and to keep your right knee directly over its ankle.

Then, you may either keep your hands on your hips (keeping your torso perpendicular to the floor and your shoulders level), or you may extend your arms out in a "T," with palms down, horizontal with the floor at your shoulders (lower if you have any stiffness or shoulder pain). Make your hands active by stretching your thumbs away from the palms, fingers together. Move both arms and hands equally away from center by really extending through your shoulders and elbows [Fig.133].

If you're bracing your rear foot against the wall and extending your arms, you will need to flex both of your hands at the wrist. Since you want to maintain balance in the muscles of both arms, extend the heel of your right hand out with the same amount of action as your left hand creates by pressing against the wall [Fig.134].

Hold your position, breathing evenly for two to eight breaths. Don't sink down into your right knee or hip socket. Instead, make your left arm and leg work to keep you balanced — extend your left arm actively away from you and keep the outside of your left foot pressing down into the floor and pulling up on your left arch.

WHAT YOU'LL FEEL

By activating your feet and legs, you will isolate a stretch in the forward inner thigh and groin and feel a firming of your legs and buttocks. If your arms are extended, you will feel a lengthening, firming, and strengthening of your arms. Depending on how long you hold the proper details, you can feel an acceleration of your respiration and heartbeat.

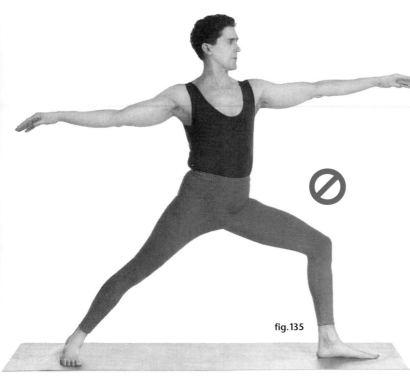

fig.135

FINE-TUNING

When you are holding your arms horizontally, be sure that you extend (activate) from the shoulders through both elbows, wrists, hands, and fingertips. Otherwise, if one or both arms are "dull" [Fig.135], the posture becomes unbalanced, heavy, and tiring, rather than exhilarating.

Hold your arms parallel to the floor. If your arms or shoulders get tired, relax your arms for a moment, then shrug your shoulders up and down before reextending your arms. But always pull your neck long, ears away from shoulders (Deer Ears). Then rotate your head to look at the fingertips of your right hand.

When you're coming up and out of the Warrior pose on your right side, test this out: try softening your left leg and arm and then come up by simply straightening your right leg. It will probably feel sluggish. You'll feel your right thigh "loading up" and getting heavy. Bend your right knee and go back down. This time before you come up, activate your left arm by extending the hand away from you. Feel as if you are extending, making space, in your left shoulder socket.

At the same time, activate your left leg by pulling up your left arch and the entire inside of your thigh while also simultaneously pressing down with your left outer heel as you straighten your right leg. Coming up should be easier.

To do the other side, simply rotate your feet 180 degrees so that they are turning toward the opposite wall. If your arms are not tired, keep them extended; if they are, bring your hands down to your hips. If you're using the wall, step your right foot in and walk your feet to the center. Stand in Mountain pose for a moment, then turn around so that your right heel is braced against the baseboard, left foot out.

Do both sides two to four times, holding each side for two to eight deep and even breaths. When you're finished, walk both feet into the center. Relax your arms as you stand in the Mountain pose, take some long, deep, smooth breaths. As you stand quietly, observe whether your respiratory or cardiovascular system has accelerated. Has your body temperature increased? If you are doing this correctly, you should feel that you have challenged yourself without feeling that you have abused your body.

► Tight

Stand in the middle of the room [Fig.132] or brace your left heel against a wall [Fig.134]. The angle of your forward knee will not be very deep. Make sure your knee does not rotate inward or beyond your ankle, which are common errors. Your stance will be fairly narrow, just about four feet. Hands begin on hips and then extend as you become more comfortable in the pose. The left hip comes forward as much as necessary so you can stabilize the right knee over its ankle and the right groin does not hurt. Be sure that the rear foot turns in, not out.

► Moderate

Stand in the middle of room [Fig.133, with your arms extended] or with your rear foot braced against a wall [Fig.134]. Your stance is moderate, from four to four and a half feet apart, depending upon the length of your legs. Your lunge is lower, but your forward knee always is directly over its ankle. Begin with your left hip slightly forward. Then slowly squeeze the left hip back, making sure to keep your right knee directly over its ankle. You'll feel more stretch in your groin.

► Flexible

Stand in the middle of the room or with your rear foot braced against a wall. Take a wide stance, up to four and a half feet apart (or wider if your legs are long). Your right knee bends close to or into a 90-degree angle and is held stable directly over its ankle. Your shoulders are down and relaxed, arms are extended, and hips are pressing toward parallel [Fig.136].

C A U T I O N

As with the Triangle, if you feel any pain in your front knee, come out of the posture, then go back down activating your feet and legs more, especially the rear leg and foot. If you still experience discomfort, narrow your stance, allow your rear hip to come farther forward, or discontinue until another day.

If you're in the middle of the room (or against the wall) and feel your feet sliding, use a sticky mat. Remember, though, that if your feet slide you may not be sufficiently activating your feet.

◄ Feet active ►

fig.136

Extended Angle Pose

The Extended Angle pose combines elements of both the Triangle and Warrior poses.

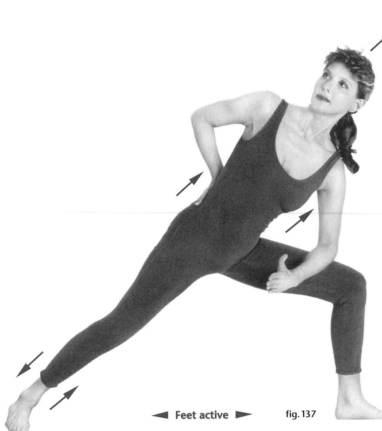

◄ **Feet active** ►   fig. 137

Begin with the Mountain pose. With your feet parallel, step them equidistantly, as wide as you did in the Warrior pose, four to four and a half feet apart, slightly wider the more flexible you are. If you did the Triangle and Warrior with your heel braced against the wall, use it now.

    Turn both feet to the right as you did for the Triangle and Warrior: right foot 90 degrees out, left foot in about half that amount. Make sure you have as much weight on your back leg as you have on the front. Now, get into the Warrior pose by slowly bending your right leg, making sure the knee comes directly over its ankle. If you're extremely flexible, the leg will form a right angle. If you are less flexible, it will not. Look down and see if your knee is lined up with your ankle. If not, adjust. At this point, your arms can be either extended as in the Warrior pose or simply on your hips.

    Now, keeping your legs stable, slowly place your right forearm on your right thigh,

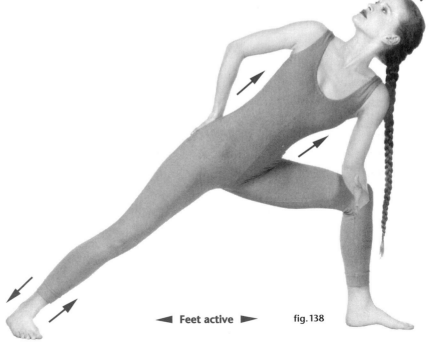

◄ **Feet active** ►   fig. 138

almost to the knee, by rotating down at your hips [Fig.137]. As you go down, feel as if you have rotated just as you did in the Triangle, from the pelvis, and that you have not allowed the right side of your torso to collapse. To do this you must move your left hip slightly forward. When your right forearm is on your thigh, activate that hand by extending the fingers long and the thumb away from the palm. Place your left hand in the small of your back, pressing it firmly.

Slowly open up your chest by rotating your left shoulder back toward the wall behind you. You will sense your chest opening wider. Keep your neck and head pulling long (Deer Ears). You can either look straight ahead or turn your head toward the ceiling and look over your left shoulder [Fig.138].

When you're ready to exit the pose, first come up into the Warrior (with arms extended or on your hips) by rotating from your hips (not just your shoulders) while pressing your left heel down. Gently use your right arm to push off your leg and help you up, if you need to. Then, slowly straighten your right knee and come to center. (Did you remember to activate your left side while coming up as you learned in Fine-Tuning on page 132?).

Switch the position of your feet. If you're working in the middle of the room, keep your legs wide and simply rotate both feet; the left will now be pointing 90 degrees to the left side and your right foot will be turned halfway in. If you've been working against the wall, step your right foot in and walk your feet together. Stand in the Mountain pose for a moment, then turn around, walk your feet apart, and press your right heel against the wall, repeating the pose on the other side.

Practice the pose, alternating sides, until you've done two to four repetitions on each side, holding each two to eight long, deep, even breaths.

C A U T I O N

If you have knee problems, take extra care not to hyper-extend (lock) your rear knee. If you feel any pain in your front knee, exit the posture, narrow your stance, then go back down. If it still hurts, activate your feet and legs more. If you still experience pain, support your rear foot against the wall or come out of the pose until another day.

If you're in the middle of the room (or against the wall) and feel your feet sliding, use a sticky mat. Remember, sliding feet may mean that you are not sufficiently activating and pulling up the arches of your feet.

WHAT YOU'LL FEEL

If you're doing this correctly, you'll be able to isolate a stretch in the forward inner thigh and groin and feel a firming of your legs and buttocks. By doing the more advanced variations you will also feel a lengthening and firming of arms and torso and depending on how assertively you practice, you may feel an acceleration of your respiration and heartbeat.

▶ **Tight**
Your stance will be narrow (about three and a half feet). Your right forearm stays on your thigh keeping the right hand active. The left hand stays pressing in the small of the back. Keep your forward knee over your ankle regardless of how far down you are. If you feel any strain, simply narrow your stance [Figs. 137 or 138].

▶ **Moderate to Flexible**
For both of these body types, the stance will be wide, about four to four and a half feet apart. Moderates, keep your right arm on your thigh for now; if you're Flexible, or can do this without straining, bring your fingertips to the floor just to the outside of your right ankle. For both types, your left hand starts in the small of the back. Once

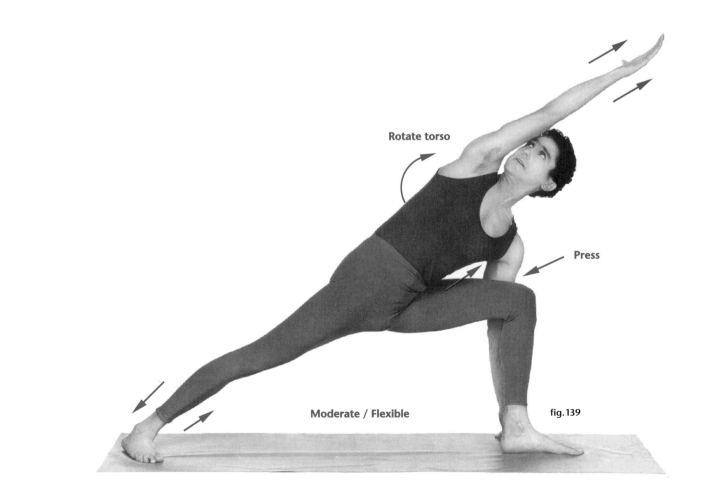

Rotate torso

Press

Moderate / Flexible

fig. 139

you're stabilized, stretch your left arm overhead and rest your left biceps lightly on your left eyebrow. Then turn your head up to look under your arm, keeping shoulder blades wide [Fig.139]. Keep your forward knee over its ankle regardless of how far down you are.

Now you can "challenge" the Extended Angle by firmly grounding the outside of your left foot and activating your left hand. Create a smooth line of energy that flows from your hips up through your entire torso through the fingertips of your left hand and from your hips down through the outside edge of your left foot. Do not drop or curve your body or arm as the dotted line shows [Fig.140].

When you're comfortable with your fingertips down, you can increase the action of the pose by "challenging" your right arm into your right knee. Press your arm into your right knee and with the same effort, press your right knee into your arm without actually moving either.

FINE-TUNING

Even though I can easily do the standing poses in the middle of the room, I often practice them with my rear heel braced against the wall. This helps "reeducate" my leg muscles to stay balanced and my spine to lengthen maximally.

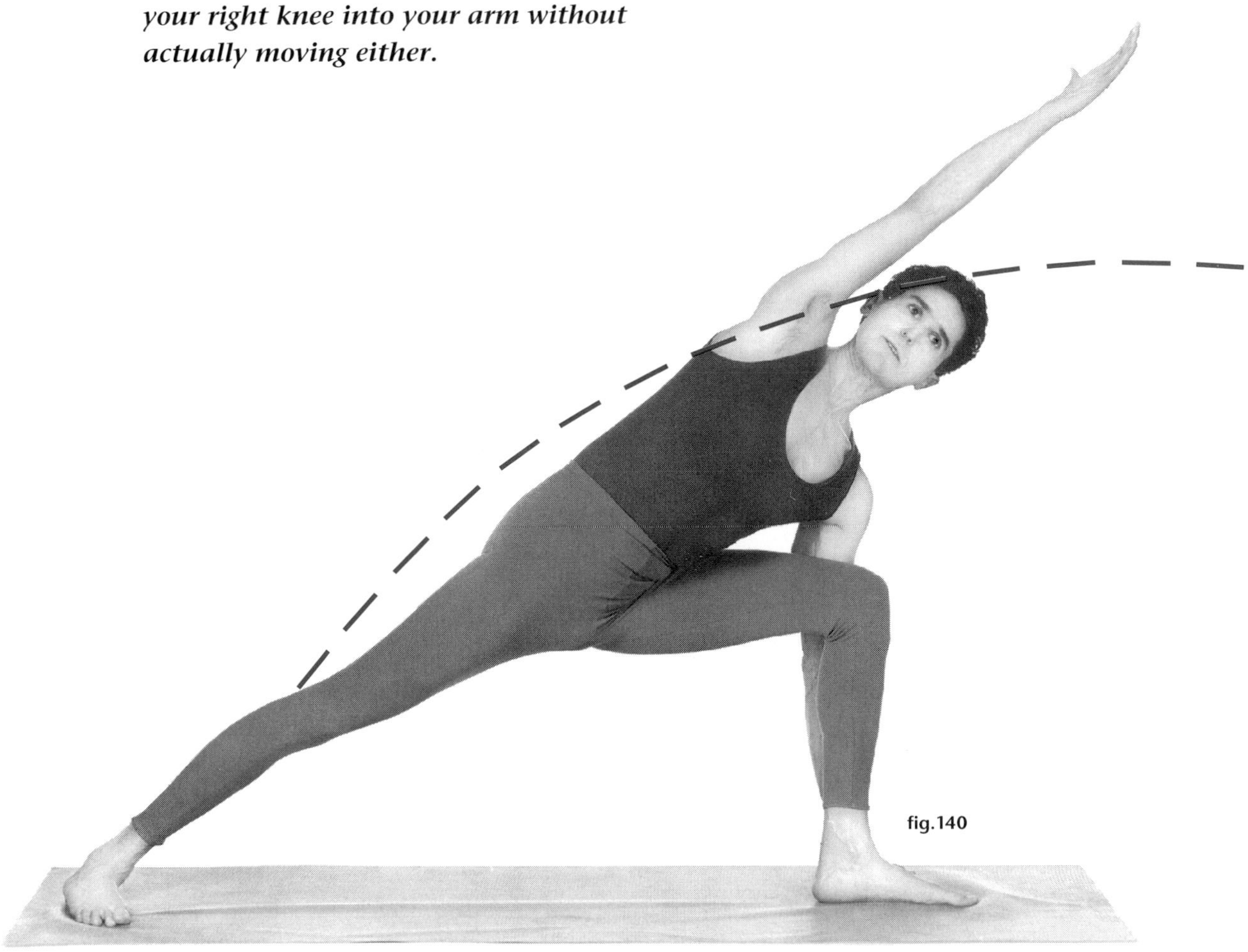

fig.140

FLOOR EXERCISES

Floor work in yoga exercise spans a wide range of movements; in the ExTension program, you'll learn a shoulder stand using a wall for support, a bridge, an exercise for your gluteal (buttocks) muscles, a stretching side twist, and a relaxation routine.

Before You Start

The floor exercises are best done on a firm (not shag) carpet. If you have a bare floor, you may want to lie on an area rug or a carpet sample, cut in a segment slightly longer than your height and about two to three feet wide, but it should not be particularly thick or soft.

For the Shoulder Stand Against the Wall, you'll need to find a clear space along a wall or a closed door, against which you can put your feet (soap and water will take care of any footprints). For the Side Twist, have a couple of firm pillows, several firm folded blankets, or two to three folded commercial carpet samples ready.

For the Relaxation pose, if your neck or chest is tight (your eyes came up above your chin while you were lying on your back), you'll need either a large folded towel, a folded blanket, or a folded piece of commercial carpet sample between one and three inches thick to place under your head.

Shoulder Stand Against the Wall

Say the word "yoga," and one of the images that always comes to mind is that of people blissfully standing on their heads and swearing that they can think better, sleep better, and digest food better. Although these claims have some validity, few of us will ever become regular head-standers. You wouldn't want to. Without proper training and a whole lot of foundation building, standing on your head can be extremely compressive and dangerous to your neck and spine.

But there is definite benefit to doing inversion exercises. For ages, it has been said that a yoga inversion practice reverses the effects of gravity, brings blood to your head for a flush of rejuvenation, thereby "nourishing the brain," takes pressure off your back and organs, increases circulation, reduces sagging skin, and promotes a deep sense of relaxation. You can do all of this without ever standing on your head. Instead, you can practice an adaptation of the Shoulder Stand Against the Wall.

CAUTION

If you have high blood pressure, hypertension, glaucoma, or a detached retina, do not do the completed Shoulder Stand Against the Wall, as it may elevate pressure in the head and eyes. Do not roll your hips up off the floor. Instead, stop when you have taken your legs up the wall and your back remains on the floor. See Appendix II, pages 178–179, for a further explanation.

Menstruating women should not do the complete Shoulder Stand Against the Wall, because the prolonged inversion has been known to cause pooling of the menses, which could lead to cramping and possible infection. The alternative postures on page 148 reduce menstrual cramps by stretching and relaxing groin and uterine tissues.

The Shoulder Stand has been called the "mother of all yoga postures" because of its nurturing feeling and effects. Practice this exercise regularly, and you will soon experience some amazing benefits. As your strength and endurance build, you will experience a profound sense of well-being because your mind feels much quieter and more relaxed. You may notice that, because of the deep, full breathing you can do in the position against a wall, congestion of the nose and chest from colds, flu, or hay fever is reduced. You will also experience increased balance as you become more confident in the pose.

Before You Start

Remember the principle I taught you in the Introduction; that *extension releases tension*. This principle is put to very good use in this Shoulder Stand, and you need to test it again before you begin.

Lie down on your back, arms along your sides. Check your head position, and if your eyes are below the level of your chin, put a folded towel, blanket, or carpet sample under your head.

Lift your left leg off the floor about six to nine inches and hold it there, allowing the foot to remain passive [Fig.141, leg soft, Fig.142, foot soft]. Notice how it starts to feel heavy, fatiguing your leg and possibly your hip. Now let it down. Try it again, but this time, as you lift your leg, extend through both your heel and the ball of your foot, as if you were pushing against a wall with your entire foot, and activating your entire leg [Fig.143, leg active, Fig.144, foot active]. Just flexing the heel isn't enough; you have to flex both the heel and the ball of your foot to keep an even extension and action in the front and back of your leg.

As you maintain your leg extension, notice that your leg doesn't get as tired as quickly and feels much more energized. Extension releases tension. Whenever you're ready, lower your leg and test this out with the other leg. Then relax and get ready to learn the Shoulder Stand Against the Wall.

C A U T I O N

Read the remainder of this section completely before proceeding. Note that the entire description for the Shoulder Stand Against the Wall sequence is first explained (and demonstrated by Susan) showing the Tight adaptation. Everyone, regardless of flexibility, should learn this entire sequence; then, if appropriate, move along to the Moderate/Flexible adaptation, which is shown in abbreviated detail.

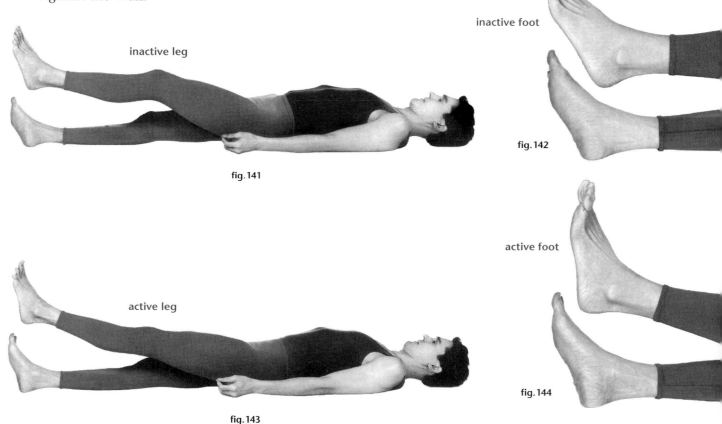

inactive leg

fig.141

inactive foot

fig.142

active leg

fig.143

active foot

fig.144

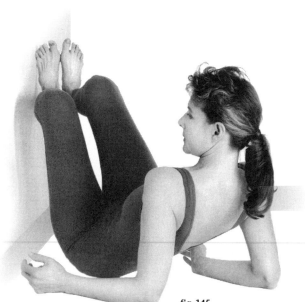

fig.145

Preparation

Find a clear wall or a closed door (make sure it's locked), and sit sideways to it [Fig.145]. If you tend to be tight (especially in the hamstrings), sit about 12 to 18 inches away. If you tend to be more flexible, sit closer to it.

Now lie back, turn so that your torso is perpendicular to the baseboard, and stretch your legs right up the wall. Be sure to *activate* both the heels and ball mounts of your feet. Let your arms stay at your sides on the floor. Your body will almost form an "L" [Fig.146]. Do *not* use a support under your head for the Shoulder Stand Against the Wall even if your eyes are below the level of your chin.

Before going any further, relax here for a moment and notice how this position feels. With your hand, make sure that your tailbone is firmly on the floor and your back has a slight arch in it. If not, you have to move slightly away from the wall. If you can move in closer to the wall without your tailbone riding up or your hamstrings hurting, do that now. Can you now feel an isolated stretch directly in the belly of both hamstrings?

Next, keep your left leg stretching up the wall with your knee *slightly* bent. Bend your right knee and put your foot flat against the wall next to your left knee. Flex your left foot and create an isolated stretch in your left hamstring by extending through your left heel and drawing down your left sitting bone [Fig.147]. If you feel more of the stretch behind your knee, slowly bend the knee more until the stretch is isolated in the belly of the hamstring. This is the same variation used in Appendix III. Repeat with the other leg.

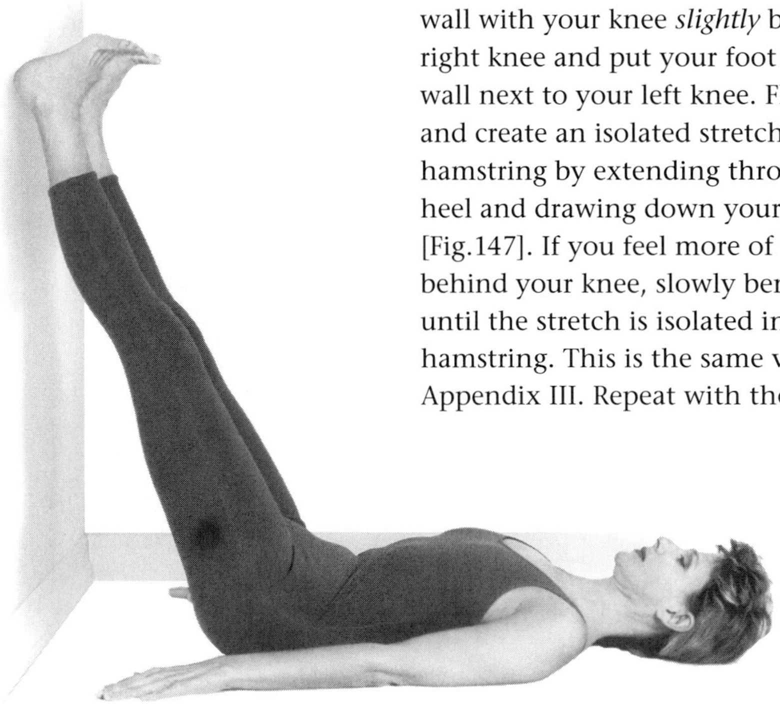

fig.146

Practice Note

Any variation of legs up the wall is a superb stretch, especially for people with low back pain, which is usually caused — or exacerbated — by tight hamstrings. It also helps to relieve tension in your hips, gluteals, neck, and shoulders. Relax up against the wall after a long day of sitting or being on your feet or any time you feel fatigued. Stay there as long as you like.

You might notice that your legs begin to tingle as you stay awhile. This is normal. Come down if and when they tingle. But as you continue to practice, you'll notice that it takes longer and longer for your legs to tingle. This is an indicator that you are subtly enhancing your endurance.

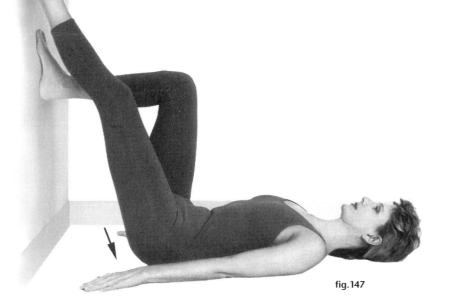

fig. 147

The Exercise

Now let's move into the Shoulder Stand Against the Wall. Begin by sitting against the wall and extending both legs up. Bend your knees (roughly 90 degrees) and put your flat feet on the wall. Slowly tilt your hips up by rolling one vertebra at a time up and off the floor, starting with your tailbone. Make this a controlled upward tilt initiated from the pubis rather than by just by lifting your hips [Fig. 148]. *As you are slowly rolling up,* you must lift your head and put it back down once or twice to release tension from your neck [Fig.149].

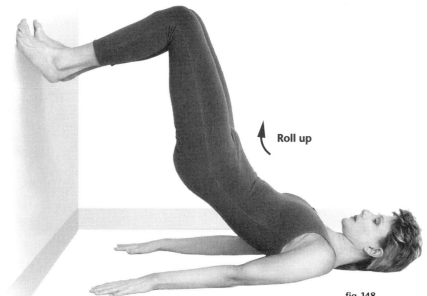

Roll up

fig. 148

Lift head and put it down several times as you roll up

fig. 149

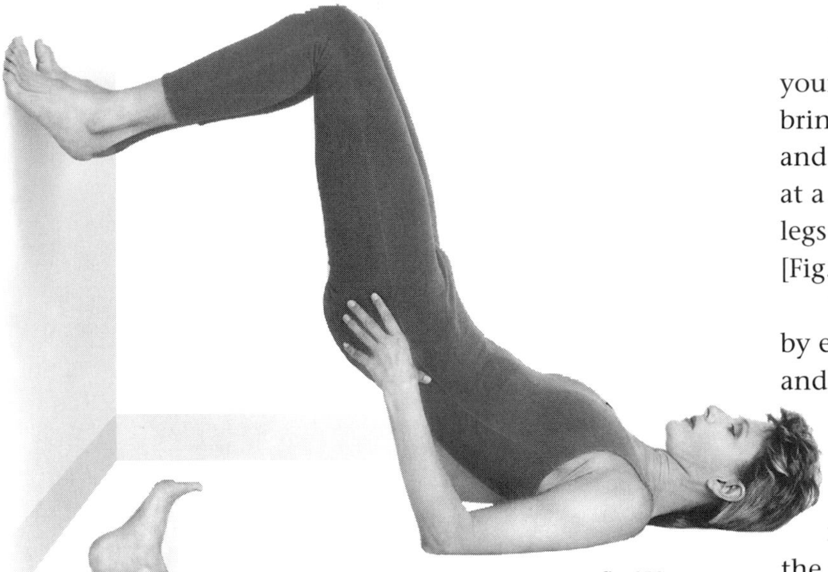

fig.150

fig.151

fig.152

Once your hips are all the way up, put your hands under them for support [Fig.150], bringing your elbows shoulder width apart and keeping them on the floor. Then, one leg at a time [Fig.151], using your heels, walk your legs all the way up the wall as far as you can [Fig.152].

When your legs are straight, activate them by extending equally through the ball mounts and heels of your feet. Make your whole body straight and firm like a board, extending strongly from your base — your shoulders — through the balls and heels of your feet. Strive to maintain a balance between the effort of the muscles in the front and those in the back of your legs.

Keep extending assertively through both the heels and ball mounts of your feet [Fig. 152]. Use your hands to push your hips up and away from your shoulders, which helps to lengthen your spine. You'll find it much easier to breathe and talk — and much more comfortable overall — if you stay active, lengthening your legs, as pressure remains *off* your neck and circulation to your head is unrestrained.

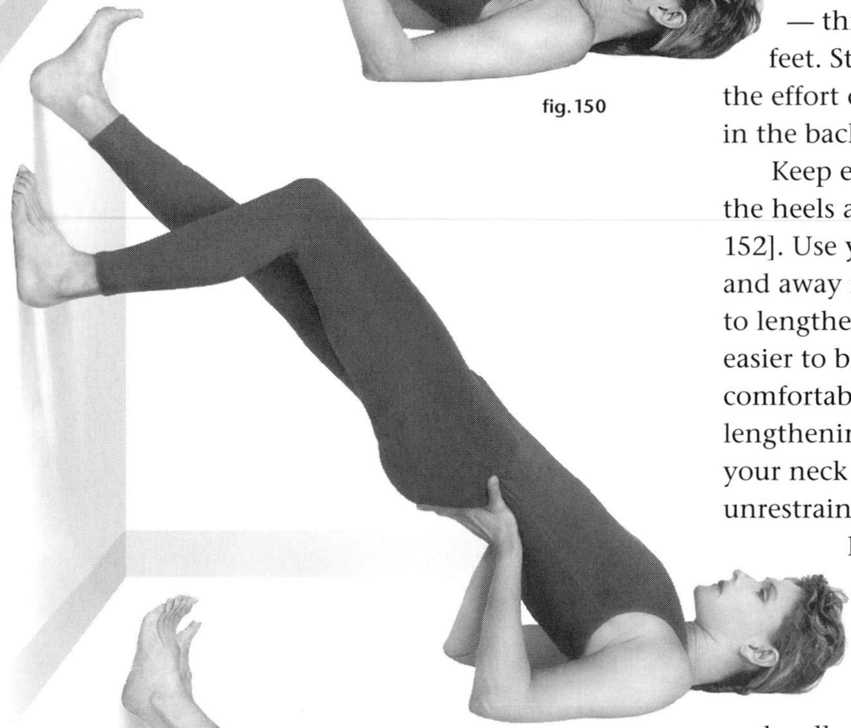

Hold the Shoulder Stand Against the Wall for five to ten long, deep breaths, longer if you can hold the extension through your legs and feet. When you're ready, bend your knees and walk your feet down the wall just as you came up [Figs.151, 150, 148, and 146], rolling down one vertebra at a time. Then relax with your legs up against the wall [Fig.146]. If you want, open your legs up wide to stretch your inner thighs [Fig.153]. Bring them back together, bend your knees again and roll over to your right side. Take a moment and breathe deeply, then slowly roll up and sit for a few moments before you continue on (as a beginner, you might experience a little light-headedness if you sit or stand up too quickly).

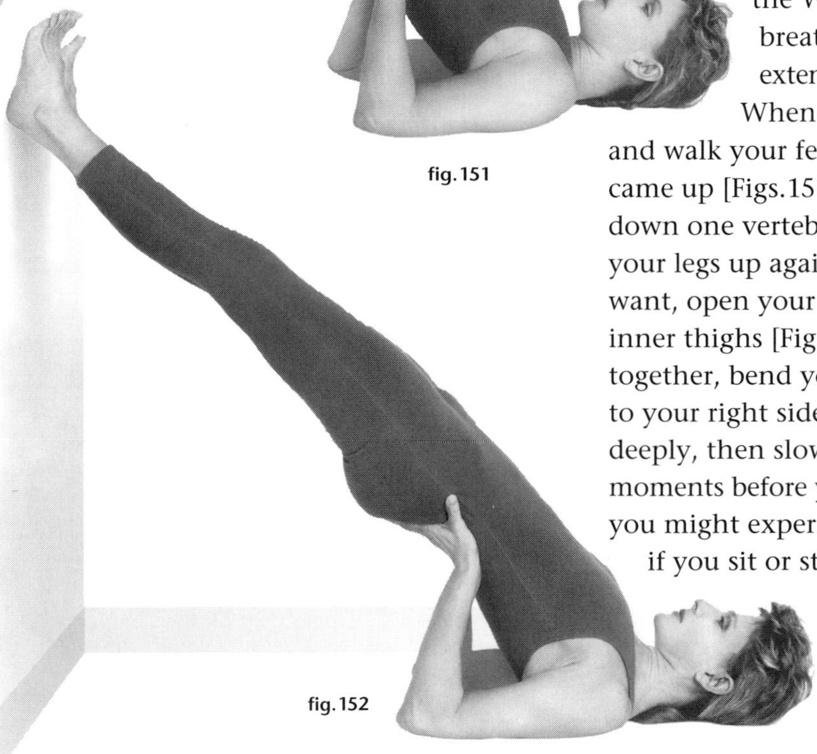

► *Tight*

Start by sitting at least a foot away from the wall; once your legs are up, feel your lower back with your hand. If you can't keep your tailbone on the floor when your legs are up, you need to scoot farther from the wall until your tailbone stays down and your lower back can maintain a natural arch. As your hamstrings become more flexible, experiment with coming closer to the wall. If you can't feel a good hamstring stretch with both legs against the wall, stretch one leg at a time up the wall [Fig.147].

Then, as you roll up, be sure to remember to lift your head once or twice and to release it back down.

► **Moderate to Flexible**

Start by sitting closer to the wall (anywhere from nine inches away to right up against it) [Fig.154]. Once your legs are up the wall, experiment with coming closer or farther (making sure your tailbone stays

FINE-TUNING

The object while in the top position of the Shoulder Stand Against the Wall is to extend your legs with sufficient energy that the base of your neck actually comes off the floor.

fig. 153

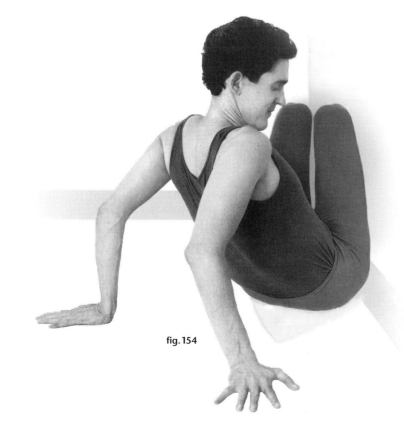

fig. 154

CAUTION

Do not turn your head from side to side while in this Shoulder Stand. If you need to see something in the room, just come down (remember to roll down vertebra by vertebra).

As a beginner, do not abruptly sit or stand up because you are likely to feel lightheaded (this phenomenon soon passes with regular practice). Instead, just slowly roll to your side, rest a moment, then slowly sit up. Rest a moment longer before you stand up.

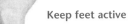

Keep foot active

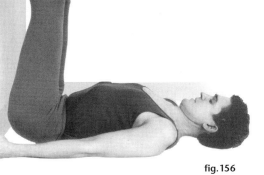

fig. 155

Keep feet active

fig. 156

Keep feet active

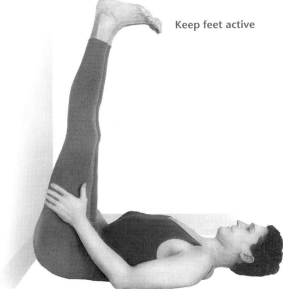

fig. 157

down). *Stretch one leg at a time up the wall, slightly bending the upward leg if necessary to isolate the stretch in the hamstrings [Fig. 155]. If your hamstrings feel tight or you feel a stretch behind the knee while your leg is straight, bend your knee just enough to isolate the stretch in the belly of the hamstrings [Fig. 156]. But if your hamstrings are so flexible that you don't feel any stretch while your legs are up against the wall, then pull them off the wall, always keeping your tailbone moving down as you point your heels [Fig. 157].*

Now, bend your knees, place both feet flat against the wall, and start the slow process of rolling upward [Fig. 158]. Remember to lift and lower your head once or twice while rolling up [Fig. 159]. Place your hands on your low back and squeeze your elbows toward each other as you walk up the wall one leg at a time [Fig. 160]. Once up the wall, be sure to keep your legs active [Fig. 161]. Adhere to the details when coming down, remembering to roll, not drop, down.

Attitude Adjustment

▶ *Aggressive*

Be sure that you have positioned your body no closer to the wall than your body type comfortably allows. **Trying to get closer to the wall will only place more stress on your neck.** *Be sure to keep your legs active and be sure to come down as soon as your legs begin to shake or when you can no longer extend fully through the legs and feet. Do not be misled by the quiet feeling this posture gives you. Although you might feel that you are wasting your time "hanging out" against the wall, there is a lot going on physiopsychologically.*

▶ *Moderate and Easygoing*

*Same as above except after rolling up, challenge yourself by staying longer. Stay for a few breaths just **after** your legs begin to shake. Then slowly roll down.*

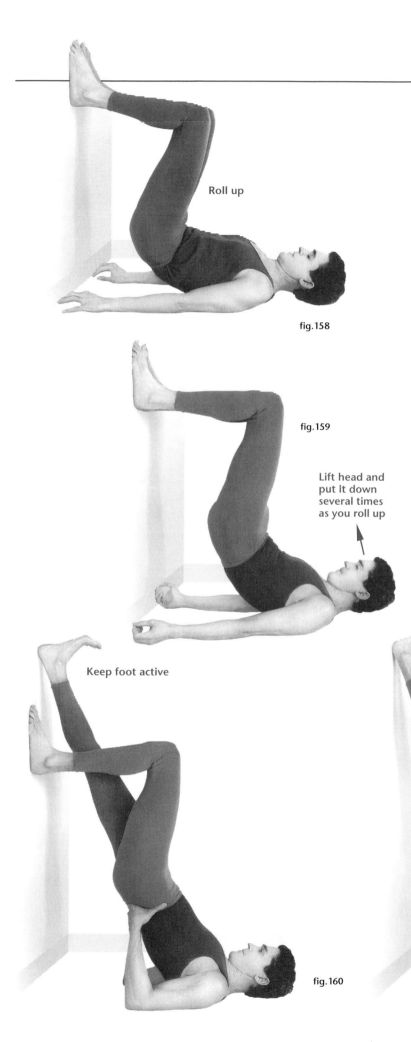

Roll up

fig.158

fig.159

Lift head and put It down several times as you roll up

Keep foot active

fig.160

Keep feet active

fig.161

WHAT YOU'LL FEEL

When you're correctly doing the preparation for the Shoulder Stand Against the Wall, you'll feel an isolated stretch in your hamstrings (either with one leg bent or with both legs extended).

As you slowly rotate up, initiating the action from the pubis, you need to feel your thigh muscles working. If you do not feel your thighs, then you are not sufficiently lifting from the pubis.

After coming up, if you're extending correctly through your legs, you'll feel equal extension along the front and back of your legs and along your spine. Your breathing will not be inhibited, and you'll be able to talk easily. There should be space between the back of your neck and the floor (if you are too close to the wall or if you are not extending properly, the back of your neck will be squished into the floor). Your neck should feel fairly free, your legs active.

Emotionally and physically, you will experience a profound sense of well-being which you can use to quiet an overactive mind and reduce emotional or physical fatigue.

Shoulder Stand Variation for Menstruating Women

Many of my women students have found that this variation provides some measure of relief from menstrual cramping.

Follow the directions to prepare for the Shoulder Stand Against the Wall except that you won't be rolling up. Once your body is in the "L" position, open your legs wide, keeping your tailbone down, and relax into the stretch [Fig. 162]. Point your heels away from you. You'll feel a stretch all along your inner thighs. Just stay there and breathe for a minute, longer if you like.

Then bring the soles of your feet together. The object is not so much to push your knees toward the wall as to press your feet together and extend your knees away from center. This should give you a nice active stretch from your groin to your knee [Fig. 163]. Hold for about a minute or longer if you have the time, deep breathing throughout. Slowly bring your legs back together; bend your knees into your chest and roll over to your side. After a few moments, sit back up.

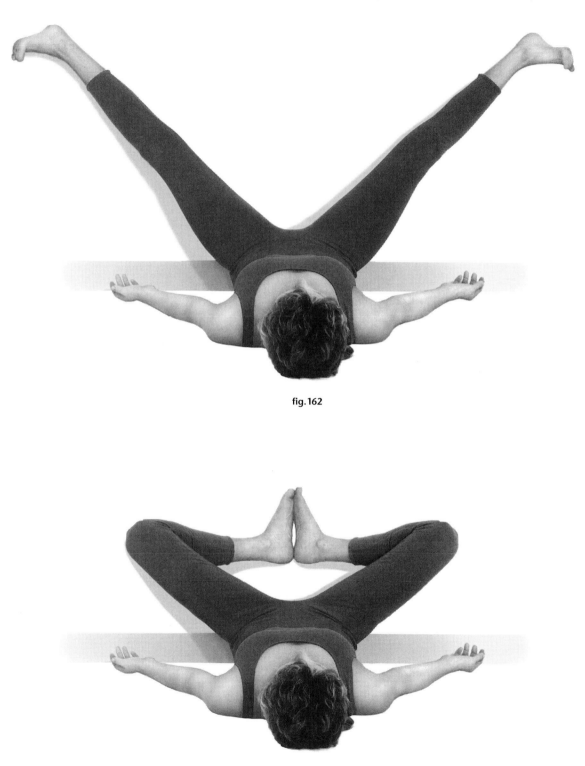

fig. 162

fig. 163

The Bridge

Research is showing that to keep your back healthy it should be strengthened and stretched. The Bridge does both. Because of the pelvic tilt up and the activation of your feet, your thighs will be toned almost magically. The pose also helps expand your breathing by stretching the muscles of your chest. It's an excellent first exercise if you've just had a baby. And the Bridge, like the Shoulder Stand Against the Wall, when practiced regularly, will leave you with feelings of emotional well-being and internal calm.

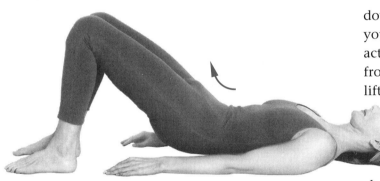

fig.164

Start on your back, hands by your sides, knees bent, feet flat on the floor, parallel and six to twelve inches apart [Fig.164]. Do *not* use a support under your head for the Bridge even if your eyes are below the level of your chin.

First, ground your feet by really pressing down with your inner and outer heels and your inner and outer ball mounts, which will activate your quadriceps (the muscles of your front thighs). Now inhale, and as you exhale, lift your pubic bone *just a little* by slowly rolling your pelvis upward. Don't come up too high; it's a very small movement known as a pelvic tilt.

fig.165

Look at Figure 165, which clearly shows the pelvic tilt. Maintain the pelvic tilt and slowly roll up — one vertebra at a time off the floor, starting with your tailbone — until you come up as far as you can [Fig.166] without feeling compression in your back. As a beginner, you can gently squeeze your buttocks together to assist the feeling of pelvic tilting.

Always keep your knees apart about the

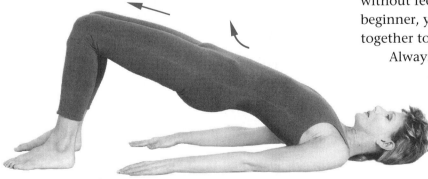

fig.166

same distance as your feet, but create a feeling of squeezing them toward each other without actually moving them. The more you activate your feet and quadriceps, the more your spine will lengthen. And lengthening your spine during the Bridge allows you to breathe deeper and keeps that compressive feeling out of your back and neck.

Do not allow your feet or knees to turn out [Fig. 167, incorrect turnout] but keep your feet active and your knees parallel maintaining a feeling that they are squeezing together [Fig. 168, correct knees and feet]. If the pose is done correctly, you will feel it almost exclusively in the tops of your thighs.

You may keep your hands at your sides or put them under your hips to support your pelvis. But don't let your hands hold you up; your thighs should be doing that. And *do not* overarch your back up.

Hold the Bridge for two to six long, easy breaths, keeping your quads and feet active. Keep your shoulders and neck relaxed by gently and slowly turning your head a little bit from side to side.

When you're ready to come down, gently reverse the process, letting down one vertebra at a time by keeping the pubis lifting when coming down. This will keep your spine extending. Remember Principle #6?

Lengthening your spine lets you breathe more freely, it enhances the stretch you feel, and helps your circulation and digestion. If you compress your spine, or slump, these processes become restricted.

Control the movement all the way down. Then relax. Go up and down two to six times, breathing deeply throughout.

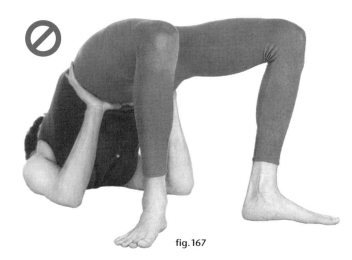

fig. 167

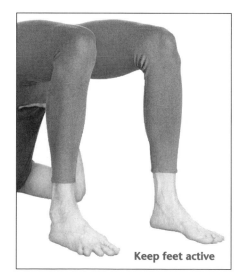

Keep feet active

fig. 168

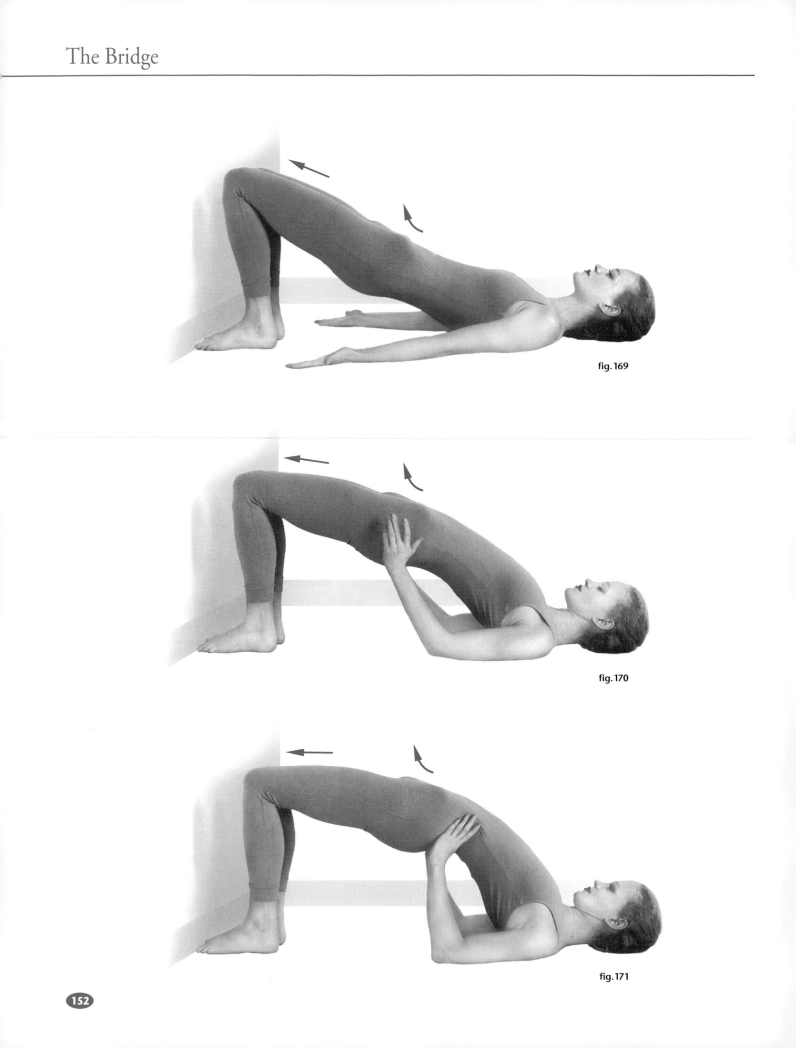

fig. 169

fig. 170

fig. 171

▶ Tight

[See sequence in Figs. 164, 165, and 166]. Your posture will be low, your lower back about six to eight inches off the floor. Your feet will be farther away from your buttocks and wider apart the first few times you practice. If you feel uncomfortable keeping your feet parallel, turn them out slightly. But as you continue to practice, bring them back toward parallel as long as there is no back or knee pain. Hips and pubic bone assertively lift, but again, not necessarily very high. Toes can be braced against the wall if you feel your feet slipping or if you feel that your legs or back need additional support as in figure 169.

▶ Moderate to Flexible

You will come up higher, with your lower back eight to twelve inches off the floor. Feet are closer to buttocks, four to ten inches apart, knees and feet parallel. Toes may be braced against the wall if you feel your feet slipping or if your legs and back need support. Although you may keep your hands on the floor [Fig. 169], it's easier to help your hips stay up if you place your hands on the sides of your hips [Fig. 170], or if you have enough flexibility, to place them directly under your lower back for support [Fig. 171]. But if you do support your hips and back, don't get lazy and let your hands do the work of holding you up. Keep your pelvis lifting and your feet and thighs active.

WHAT YOU'LL FEEL

If you're doing the Bridge correctly — maintaining the squeeze in your thighs and buttocks — you'll feel a pleasant "working" of your quadriceps and gluteal muscles. Your spine will feel long, without tightness in your lower back. Your breath will be long and free, your head will not feel heavy, and your face will not redden. Practice regularly and you'll be amazed at how strong and firm your thighs and buttocks will become.

FINE-TUNING

If you feel any knee pain, first try pressing the inner ball and heel of both feet more assertively into the floor while simultaneously lifting your arches and squeezing your knees toward center without actually moving them. If that doesn't work, experiment with your foot placement by moving your feet wider or closer together; or try turning your toes in or out just a little — not as far as Figure 167. If your knee(s) still continues to hurt, come down, rest, and try again, this time with your feet farther away from your buttocks. Another alternative to releasing knee pain is to do the Bridge with your toes against a wall for additional support [Fig. 170].

Gluteal Rolling

This is one exercise you probably won't see in many exercise classes.
I encourage students to do it at any time during class when they feel tired or need a break. And I always have everyone do it near the beginning and end of each class. It helps to restore tone and flexibility to your gluteal muscles (and hip rotators). And that means better-looking buttocks.

Sit on the floor. Bend and bring your knees toward your chest as close as is comfortable and lean back on your right hand or elbow and forearm. Activate your feet by flexing them up and extending through both the heels and ball mounts.

Now, roll on your right buttock by drawing your knees in and then around in a circle [Figs.172 and 173]. Make the circle wide enough that the entire gluteal area is massaged, always keeping your knees bent. If you have back problems or feel any pain in your lower back, keep the circles small and knees closer to chest.

Roll for 20 to 60 seconds on your right side, lower your knees, then switch to the left side. Always make sure you lower your knees before switching sides to avoid rolling over your tailbone. Repeat for 20 to 60 seconds on your left side, then alternate two to four more times.

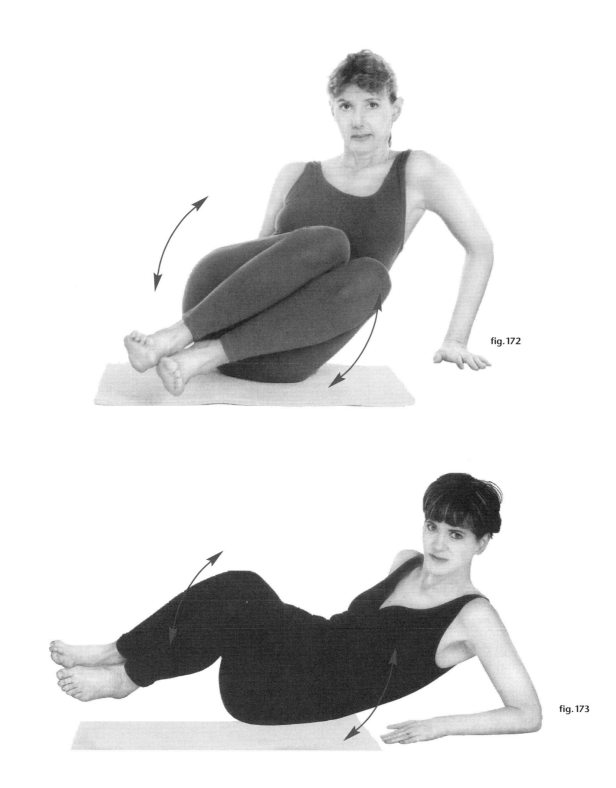

fig. 172

fig. 173

The ExTension Side Twist

The Side Twist helps relieve back stiffness and pain and helps promote better circulation to your back, abdominal, and waist muscles. It also reduces cramps and indigestion and strengthens your abdominal muscles. You've probably done it, or at least seen it done, in all kinds of exercise or rehabilitation programs. But the common way of teaching it leaves out several crucial elements, which you'll be learning: the "jog" of the hips, active hands and arms, and the palms turned up. What we've done is simply make something good even better. (If you want to experience a dramatic difference between the ExTension Side Twist and a standard Side Twist, complete this section and then turn to in Appendix II and follow the directions for the standard twist.)

CAUTION

Read this entire section before doing the ExTension Side Twist. If you are Tight (or even Moderate), be sure to have your props available and use them as instructed.

Do not do the Side Twist after abdominal, back, or chest surgery unless approved by your doctor.

Lie on your back with your knees bent, feet flat on the floor. First check your head position. If your eyes are lower than your chin, place a folded blanket or carpet sample under your head to help keep your shoulders and neck relaxed. Start with your arms extending away from your body slightly lower than your shoulders with your palms turned up and hands active [Fig. 174]. Turning your palms upward opens your chest and allows you to breathe and relax more deeply.

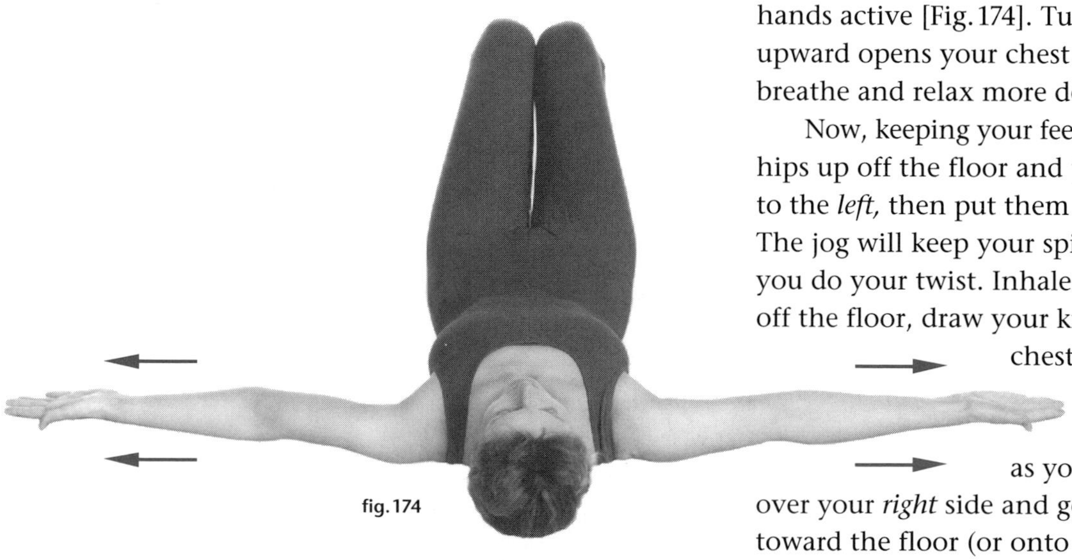

Now, keeping your feet planted, just lift your hips up off the floor and jog them significantly to the *left,* then put them back down [Fig. 175]. The jog will keep your spine in alignment as you do your twist. Inhale and, taking your feet off the floor, draw your knees toward your chest — only as far as is comfortable for your back — then, as you exhale, rotate them over your *right* side and gently let them down toward the floor (or onto props if appropriate). Keep your head looking straight up [Fig. 176].

Stop now and check a few things out. Has your left shoulder come way off the floor? Does your back hurt at all? If there is any tension at all, even just a little discomfort,

fig. 174

follow the directions for Tight. This is supposed to be a relaxing exercise, so any tension, anywhere, is counterproductive.

Stay in your twist breathing deeply for 10 to 30 seconds keeping your hands and feet active. Activate your hands by straightening your fingers and stretching your thumbs away from your palms [Fig.176]. Activate your feet by extending through the four points of your feet [Fig.177].

When you're ready, rotate back to center while exhaling (use your abdominal muscles to help you). Then plant your feet firmly, and jog your hips off center to the *right*. Bring your knees into your chest, take a deep inhalation, then exhale and gently let your knees down to the floor (or supports) to your *left*, making all the necessary adjustments.

Do the ExTension Side Twist three to twelve times going from side to side. Learn to move into your twist only on the exhalation. Stay and relax in the twist while you are inhaling.

After twisting, conclude your exercise session with the Relaxation exercise that follows.

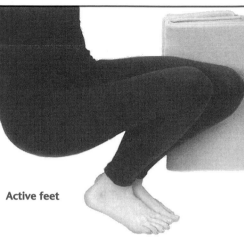

fig.177

Active feet

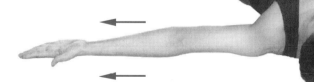

fig.175

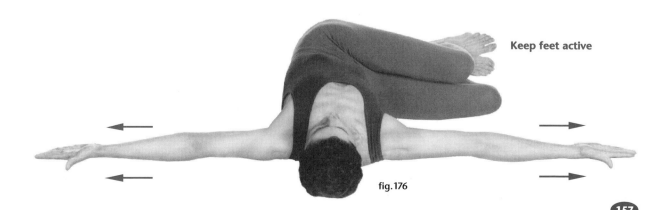

Keep feet active

fig.176

► **Tight**

Have your supports ready. Put a firm pillow, a few folded carpet samples, or a stack of firm blankets on either side of you where your knees will be when they reach the floor in your twist. Make sure they're about four to twelve inches high, more or less, depending on your level of comfort. From the starting position with your feet on the floor, jog your hips off center to left [Fig. 178]. Keep your arms lower than the level of your shoulders.

On your exhalation, twist your torso and let your knees come down to the support on your right side [Fig. 179]. If there is any discomfort at all, use a higher support or move your knees farther from your chest. If your left shoulder comes significantly off the floor, bring your arms down from the "T" until your shoulder moves closer to the floor (it's okay for it to be off the floor just a little). If it is still way off the floor, move your knees down, away from your chest a little more.

► **Moderate**

Use low or no supports. Arms should almost form a "T." Jog hips significantly to the left [Fig. 175]. Knees are bent a little higher into the chest. Then exhale as you slowly rotate knees toward the right side and down to floor [Fig. 176].

fig. 178

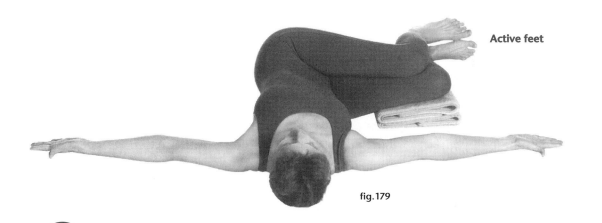

Active feet

fig. 179

▶ **Flexible**

Your arms should form a perfect "T," never higher. After jogging your hips significantly to the left, remove your feet from the floor. Take your bent knees higher and closer to your chest. Rotate down to the right on exhalation. Then with every exhalation and keeping your arms long and extended, feel as if you further rotate your torso to the left, striving to keep your spine long. Keep your hands and feet active throughout.

Advanced variation #1: If after having completed several twists to both sides and you wish a deeper twist, you may press your right arm over your top knee [Fig.180], and each time you exhale, rotate your torso a little bit more to the left.

Advanced variation #2: The stretch may be enhanced by crossing the right knee over the left knee keeping arms at a "T." Or as you cross the right knee over the left, press the right arm down over the top knee [Fig.181].

WHAT YOU'LL FEEL

The spiral effect may cause a gentle, pleasant clicking or popping in your back as your vertebrae muscles release their tightness and your spine automatically adjusts. You'll sense a stretching in your middle to lower back, obliques (the sides of your belly), abdominals, and across your chest. You shouldn't feel any tension or pain in your shoulders or neck (if you do, bring your arms lower) or pain in your back (if you do, bring your knees farther from your chest before you begin your twist and always, if your back hurts, use props).

FINE-TUNING

All twists need to have active hands, with palms up, and active feet. Your twisting will be best when you evenly activate both hands with the same energy or attention that you use when you evenly activate both feet.

When you are totally comfortable in your twist, regardless of variation, it can be enhanced by picking your head up off the floor and turning it so that you are looking at the side away from your legs. Then place your ear down on the floor maintaining that feeling of Deer Ears.

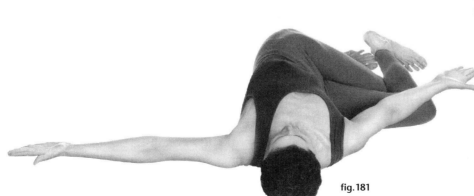
fig.180

fig.181

Relaxation

Relaxation is probably the most important aspect of this entire program.

It's the part that really does relax, release, and rejuvenate you. Yet most people find it very difficult to relax. You may think you don't really need it or don't have time for it. You may be tempted to skip it altogether. I strongly urge you not to!

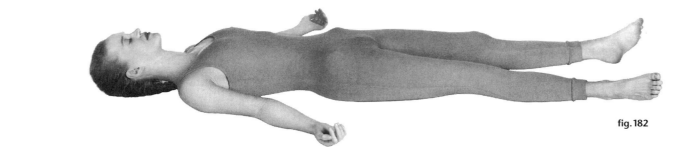

fig. 182

For every 20 minutes of exercise, you need only a couple of minutes for relaxation. The relaxation phase not only serves to help you hold on to the great feeling you've created from exercise, but it can reduce tension and hypertension and maybe even add years to your life.

During the exercise component, you are learning to actively balance the major muscles of your entire body, which ultimately quiets your mind and creates an alpha state while you exercise (refer back to Principle #8, page 29, which explains this phenomenon).

In the formal relaxation segment that follows, you'll learn how to let go of everything, how to relax your body and your mind completely to create a total quiet, relaxed physical and mental state.

To gain the most benefit in the least amount of time, it is crucial to position your body properly on the floor. If there is any tension in your body, it takes longer for it to relax, if it ever does.

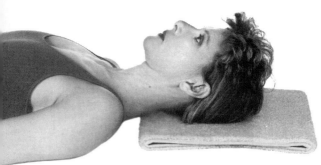

fig. 183

Preparation

You learned how to prepare for relaxation in the introduction. Lie down on your back with your legs extended, your feet about eight to twelve inches apart flopping outward, and your arms on the floor, hands about 18 inches away from your sides with palms up [Fig. 182].

While you lie in this position, scan your body. How do your neck and upper back feel? Place a folded towel or carpet sample under your head [Fig. 183]. Do your neck, head, or upper back feel better or worse with the support under your head? If there is no difference, or if it feels worse, don't use it. Now place a pillow or rolled carpet sample under your knees [Fig. 184], or put your feet and calves up on a bench, chair, or sofa with your knees bent [Fig. 185]. Does this feel any better than when your legs were flat on the floor? If there is no difference or it feels worse, don't use it.

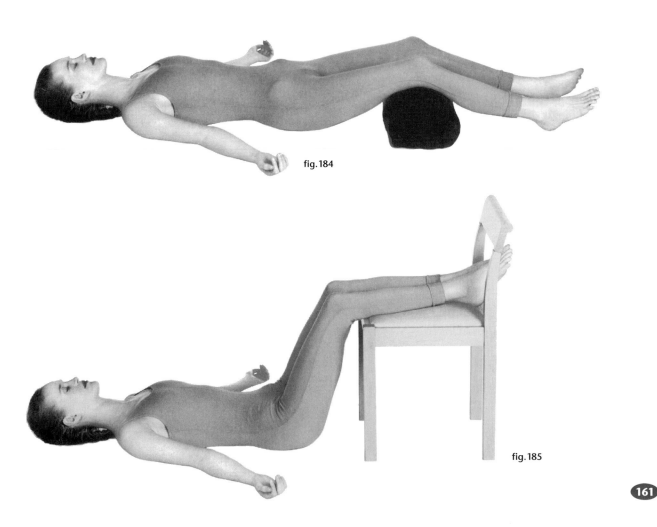

fig. 184

fig. 185

As you lie on the floor, be sure that your fingers and hands are soft, not stiff as in Figure 186. If fingers or hands are tight, the body cannot relax completely. To ensure hand softness, curl your fingers tightly into a fist, then let them open a little so that they remain softly curled [Fig.187]. Also relax your face.

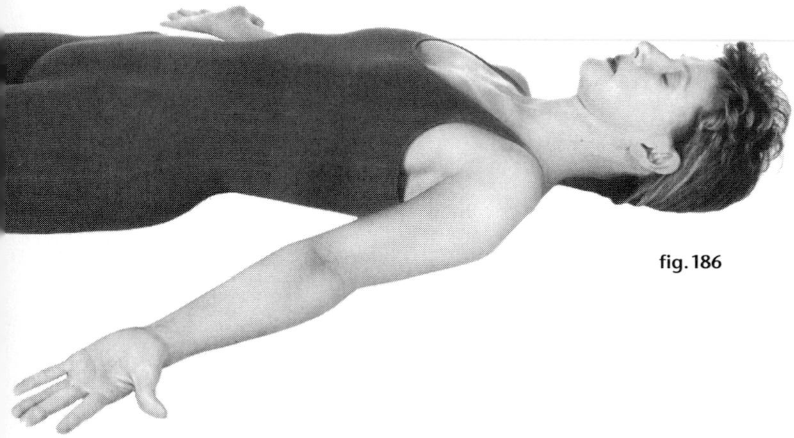

Relax

Take a few minutes to relax completely while in position. You're going to be doing a progressive relaxation, which involves tightening and releasing various muscles of your body. You'll be training yourself to recognize softness by first tensing up, then releasing. This way, you will know what relaxation really feels like. Doing this at the end of your exercise session is a great way to "seal in" the work you've done, to maintain the toning, the energy, and the relaxation. You can use these techniques, abbreviated, during the day while sitting at your desk to ease anxiety and tension, or do the full routine at night while in bed to relax you into a deep and restful night's sleep.

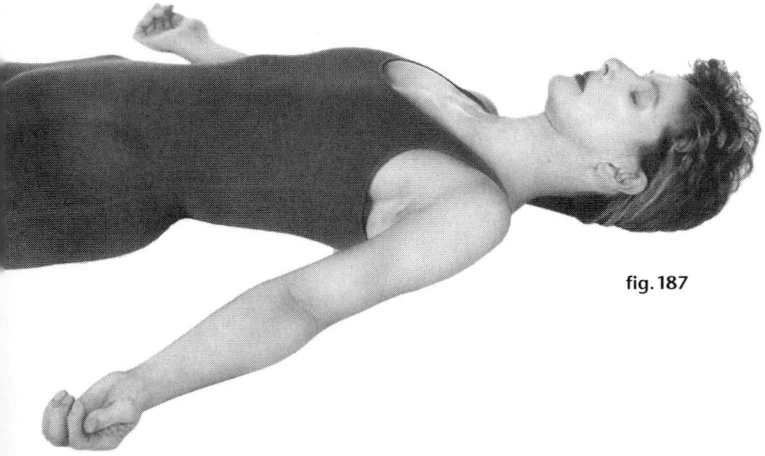

What follows is a brief description of a progressive relaxation. Read it through a few times to familiarize yourself with the process. Then simply lie down and do it. The first couple of times you practice it, you might feel as if nothing has happened. But when always done right after your ExTension exercises, you will soon begin to feel its soothing and relaxing effects.

If you'd like to talk yourself through one and you have a tape recorder, turn to Appendix IV, where you'll find a full progressive relaxation that will take you between five and ten minutes (depending upon your speaking speed and the amount of time you pause between "phrases").

fig. 186

fig. 187

Lying on the floor, in a comfortable position, take several long, soft, deep inhalations and exhalations, then relax your breath and be still for a few moments.

Start with your toes and your feet. Inhale and tighten both your toes and your feet. Hold for a moment then exhale and let them go.

Move on to your ankles and calves. Take a deep, soft inhalation and tighten both your ankles and calves. Then, exhale and let them go.

Go through your whole body, moving on to your knees, then your thighs, your buttocks, your belly, and your lower back. Move down to your hands (make a fist and squeeze), then up your arms to your shoulders, chest, and neck. Finish with your face. Tighten your jaw and your mouth, furrow your brow, then release. Each time you tighten, inhale, hold, and release with an audible exhalation.

When you've gone through your body, relax and breathe in very deeply, then let it out, letting the exhalation last longer than the inhalation. Keep breathing and imagine yourself sinking deeply down into the floor. Count to yourself from five down to the number one, and with every number that you count, relax deeper.

Just lie there and breathe for a while. When you're ready to come up, count to yourself from one back up to five, coming more awake as you count higher. When you get to five, take a deep breath, and let it out.

Slowly roll to your right side, taking your knees into your chest and relax for a moment, making a pillow with your arms so that your head is relaxed. Stay there as long as you like. Then slowly sit up into any comfortable position and remain sitting with a long spine until you are ready to get up.

At this point, your relaxation component is completed. When you are ready, you might want to come up to your hands and knees, place one foot flat underneath you, place a hand on that thigh and slowly push yourself up to standing. Go about your day feeling relaxed and rejuvenated.

PRACTICE NOTE

If you are going to be sitting for a couple of minutes, try putting something firm under your hips while sitting: one or more folded carpet samples, a firm folded blanket or two, or maybe a couple of big books. This will take pressure off your knees, hips, and back, helps keep the spine longer, and allows you to breathe deeper and easier.

PART III

CONCLUSION

Plenty of us have drifted into patterns of laziness and inactivity; most people are not sure why. I think it's because our bodies have started to change as we age, and we just don't know what to do about it.

Growing older has its advantages, of course. Experience, tolerance, relationships.

But I would be lying to you if I said that I like the physical changes. I feel tired sometimes, too. It's tempting just to do nothing.

By practicing the ExTension program, however, my body has developed an integrity, a grace, that it did not have when I was younger.

The goal of this program is to create a lifelong habit; that means changing the unconscious habits that already exist in your body. It takes some practice, and you cannot learn it by reading alone. You have to train your body. Regularly.

The beauty of ExTension is that "regularly" means an investment of only 20 minutes a day, maybe four days a week. And it means investing time in a program that is much better than both alternatives: not exercising at all or risking your pain-free body in most all other forms of aggressive and abusive exercise.

Although the exercises presented in ExTension are extremely basic, they create foundations that will help your body cope with the inevitable changes of growing older: *Strength* for everyday tasks, work, and play. *Flexibility* to keep your movement fluid and effortless. *Endurance* to keep your heart and lungs healthy. And *peace of mind* to help you weather the stresses that your life, no matter how settled, is bound to include. And those foundations will keep you looking and feeling great.

With ExTension, you can grow old gracefully. For me, it's time well spent.

To Learn More

I truly hope that you take the time to read the material in the Appendixes that follow and experience the standard way of doing the exercises. If you are like most of us who have come from traditional and standard methods of exercise and have then learned ExTension, you'll get excited about this alternative and will want to learn more.

If you are interested in learning more about the ExTension program in person, you can sponsor a weekend ExTension seminar, which would bring me to your area to conduct a foundational workshop. I'll leave you and your group with many additional exercises that will stimulate and challenge you in a nonaggressive and non-competitive environment. Contact me through my address in Resources, Appendix VI.

APPENDIX I

RELAX, RELEASE, AND REJUVENATE
FOR THE REST OF YOUR LIFE

Most people don't read the Appendix of a book. Especially an exercise book. They figure all they really need to do is do the exercises correctly, and that's it.

You could do that with this book and still reap many benefits from the ExTension program.

Or you could try something completely different and see the program as the start of a new way of moving, exercising, and living your life.

My experience as a teacher has shown me again and again that students get faster results and stay with the program longer when they understand how and why ExTension works.

You already know the basics, but there are several more elements to a deeper understanding of ExTension. First, I want you to understand more about how your body is constructed; second, how soft tissue responds to exercise and pain; and third, the role fascia plays as you grow older.

Finally, I feel that it is important for you to experience how yoga-based exercises are traditionally practiced. Then, from your own experience, you will know just how powerful and fundamentally correct ExTension is.

APPENDIX I

WHY EXTENSION WORKS

As you read in the Introduction, in the ExTension program we're concerned with four types of soft tissue — muscle, tendon, ligament and above, all, fascia — and how they all relate to the skeletal system.

In 1947, medical artist Peter Bachin developed several significant charts. One is called "The Muscular System" and shows in remarkable detail muscles and tendons. The other is "The Skeletal System," which illustrates tendons and bones and shows how your skeleton looks when the soft tissue of your body is in perfect balance both in the front and the rear of your body (the Bachin charts are in Appendix V).

The first thing I want you to understand is just what these terms mean.

The Skeleton and the Plumb Line

When you were young, your body was probably in better balance than it is now. You had no trouble standing directly upright. The strength and flexibility of the muscles in the front of your body were in near-perfect balance with those in the back of your body. Nothing pulled you forward or back. You were on the plumb.

Look again at both Bachin charts. The muscles shown in "The Muscular System" are in perfect balance, front and rear. The plumb line drawn on "The Skeletal System" runs directly through the center of the body.

Those examples are the ideal because when that balance occurs, your skeleton, not your muscles, holds your body upright. What does this mean? Stand up for a moment. Stand as straight as you comfortably can. Now lean forward, just shifting your weight forward but keeping your heels down. Stay there for a while. What do you feel in the front of your body? Bring your head a little bit farther forward. Feel the "loading up" of the muscles on the front of your shins? Your thighs? Imagine standing imbalanced like this all day long. Every day. Year after year.

Many of us do. Not intentionally, of course. You may have had an accident, or other trauma, or simply gotten used to poor posture. Whatever the cause, as imbalanced muscles chronically contract over time, the body will habituate to the discomfort of the loaded and soon to be very tight muscles. After a while, you will no longer feel the discomfort. You will simply become fatigued well before your day is over. And you won't understand why.

Well, I have a couple of theories why.

The first one is very simple: If the muscles in your body are imbalanced, and the tighter ones, say, in the front of your body are trying to overcome the weaker rear muscles, they are constantly fighting each other to keep your body erect. It's so subtle that you don't notice it, but it wipes you out.

The second is a bit more complicated: When your body is out of balance and chronically tight, it just won't absorb proper nutrition. This accelerates your fatigue and causes you to become tighter. As you find your body becoming tighter and more lethargic, it becomes more difficult to exercise and you feel even more tired. At this point, many people gain weight because they just begin taking in more calories than they expend.

This is what can happen when your body is off the plumb, when your muscles are no longer in balance. You become chronically tired; your strength, endurance, and flexibility decline. You lose your once good posture. By using ExTension as a tool, you can take active responsibility for getting yourself back on the plumb.

Muscle

Muscles move bodies. They pull on our bones and move our limbs; they pump fluids throughout our body, and through their pumping action, they make our organs work. The muscles in which we are specifically interested are the larger groups that attach to bones and move our body.

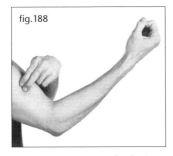
fig.188

You learned this proof during the preparation for the Forward Bend, but do it again. Bend your arm at the elbow and make a muscle. Take your other hand and squeeze that muscle right in the middle [Fig.188] (this is your biceps muscle). Notice that when you bend and straighten your arm, you can feel the biceps expand and contract. The muscle is elastic and spongy. It is pliable and is designed to be lengthened and shortened. When you look at "The Muscular System," you see that muscles are darker than tendons and ligaments. That's because they are are deeply infused with blood.

Proper circulation of blood oxygenates muscle tissue, bringing the energy and nourishment for movement, growth, and healing. Good blood circulation helps muscles work toward their endurance limits.

Do you remember feeling sore for a day or two after exercising? That soreness is a result of irritated muscle fiber as well as a buildup of lactic acid and other waste products. When you work out, you always create tiny microscopic tears in muscle fiber. But because there is so much blood circulation in muscle tissue, those micro-tears heal very quickly and the soreness dissipates.

Muscle will only contract when it has been stimulated. Under normal conditions, the brain sends a message to the muscle, stimulating it to contract. Then it releases. During normal movement, including exercise, muscle tissue alternately contracts and releases. Muscle also contracts when it has been traumatized, but when traumatized, it usually will not relax. It may stay in a state of chronic tension — and the muscle stays stimulated. This state of chronic tension saps your body's energy, and normal functioning is reduced. When this happens, muscles become chronically tired. You become tired. In addition, chronically contracted muscles pull on their attachments, and your body is pulled off the plumb.

During exercise, we want to minimize trauma to soft tissue. We want to stretch and strengthen tissue, not irritate and chronically contract it. ExTension teaches you how.

Tendon

Bend your arm again and start squeezing the muscle closer and closer to your elbow [Fig.189]. What happens to the muscle? It becomes thinner, harder, and denser. As muscle moves closer to bone, it merges into tendon. It is tendon that attaches to bone, not muscle. If you look again at "The Muscular System," you will see that muscle turns white as it merges into tendon. Just by feeling with your fingers you can tell that tendon is less spongy than muscle tissue; it doesn't have as much blood circulation as muscle. It is designed to hold, not stretch as muscle does.

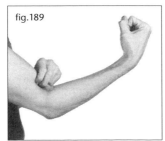
fig.189

Therefore, if tendon is overstretched or otherwise traumatized, it takes a long time to heal. This injury is called tendonitis. Tendonitis injuries are always painful and take longer to heal the older you become. In this or any other exercise program, you should avoid stretching tendon. ExTension teaches you how.

Ligament

Ligament connects bone to bone. Look at the knee detail in Bachin's "Skeleton System." It shows that ligament is completely white with virtually no blood circulation. Severe ligament injuries do not heal by themselves. They usually require surgery.

Obviously, you don't want to irritate or tear a ligament. Unknowingly, most people involved in exercise movement often stretch deep within their joints, irritating not only tendons but ligaments as well. We want to avoid deep joint and ligament stretching. ExTension teaches you how.

The All-Important Fascia

Although the Bachin charts do not show it (nor for that matter, do most anatomy books), permeating your entire body is a fourth connective tissue, called fascia. As I told you in the Introduction, fascia is the whitish, almost transparent fiber that you see when you pull the skin off a chicken breast.

You have fascia too. It covers your entire body, under your skin, from the top of your head to the tip of your toes. Fascia also surrounds every muscle fiber and all of your organs and glands (see Clemente's Anatomy in Appendix V). Fascia has been called "the bag that holds the body together." It connects everything, but has no specific, identifiable origin or insertion, as muscles have.

Although fascia is still little studied, I believe that it's involved with the stiffness and pain we experience as we grow older. And understanding fascia's mechanisms is the key to understanding how to exercise appropriately.

Physical and emotional injuries, little tweaks, micro-tears, simple pulls, and the wear and tear of daily life — all these everyday occurrences affect all of your soft tissues through the years. What happens to soft tissue when it's injured or traumatized? It contracts.

It has to. It's a way of making you slow down and allow an injury to heal while you continue to live your life. The contraction of fascia and muscle protects you from exacerbating your injuries. Unfortunately, however, after those injuries "heal" (if in fact they ever really do), contracted fascia seldom releases back to its preinjured state. You heal, but your body remembers.

I believe that as we grow older, the fascia around old injuries contracts further. Compounding that, about every ten years beginning from about the ages of 28 to 32, fascia becomes less resilient and causes the muscles it surrounds to become tighter and tighter,
which, indirectly, exacerbates preexisting injuries and pain. Have you noticed that as you go through those ten-year thresholds (28 to 32, 38 to 42, 48 to 52, and so on) you start to feel long-ago injuries again? Or perhaps at best, are you starting to feel sluggish and tighter? Why does this happen? I believe that Hilton's Law helps provide us with an explanation.

APPENDIX I

HILTON'S LAW: UNDERSTANDING FASCIA IS IMPORTANT TO UNDERSTANDING EXTENSION

Understanding Hilton's Law becomes more important especially as we pass through those ten-year increments. The law states: "The nerve root that supplies a joint, supplies all the muscles attaching to that joint, and the overlying skin."

Therefore, the nerve root must also supply the overlying fascia as it passes on to the skin. As fascia contracts, nerves are stimulated, which in turn stimulates the underlying muscles served by that nerve, which in turn stimulates the joint of that nerve (reversing Hilton's Law) thereby stimulating all other muscles that attach to the joint. And what do muscles do under stimulation? They contract. And you get tighter, and tighter, and tighter.

Let me paint you a picture of how this works. When you were young, you could "go for it" any time you wanted. You could stress and abuse your body a great deal and it responded. Sometimes there was pain, but you could work through it. Your coaches or instructors told you, "No pain, no gain." They seemed to be right. You became stronger, and your endurance grew.

But that was years ago, and you have since passed through one or more of those ten-year thresholds. It's been a while since you've exercised, but you want to begin a new stretching-exercise program. The author of the new book you just bought, or your new exercise instructor or — worse yet — your inner voice tells you to go for it and to try hard. And so you do. But you end up hurting all over your body for days afterward. You have overstretched and overexercised everything. Here's what's happened.

Your fascia has contracted during the years. When you attempted to restore your former flexibility, you became tighter. You irritated old facilitated pathways (in acupuncture terminology, a facilitated pathway develops as a result of injury which allows easy recurrence of irritation and pain). As much as you don't want to, you have to quit — again.

You went too deeply too quickly. And this is what Hilton's Law is all about. If you go too deeply too quickly, you will irritate the fascia. As the fascia is irritated, it contracts. As it contracts, the underlying muscle becomes stimulated. And so on. You end up causing contraction and lethargy, not flexibility and energy.

During my study of NeuroMuscular therapy, I found that soft tissue contraction and pain were resolved much more quickly by initially working at the level of the superficial fascia, near the surface, not by working into muscle or deep fascia. That is one of the reasons that I changed my approach to yoga exercise. I learned that doing less and working appropriate soft tissue first, I obtained quicker and safer results. Therefore, yoga exercise as I teach it in ExTension begins at the level of fascia.

That's why I tell you to avoid pain, to avoid going too deeply too quickly. Particularly as you grow older. And this is the power of ExTension. It teaches you how to exercise your body intelligently by doing less to get you more and to avoid overstimulating soft tissue until it is ready to respond.

APPENDIX II

TEST THE TRADITIONAL WAY
OF DOING THE EXERCISES

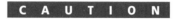

C A U T I O N

The following section shows you the more traditional way of doing some of the exercises
taught in ExTension. Some of the traditional exercises can be difficult. If you have preexisting injuries
that might be exacerbated by doing any of these exercises, don't do them.

BEFORE YOU BEGIN

Now that you have experienced the ExTension way of doing the program, I'm going to ask you to test
the standard, traditional ways of doing several of the exercises. You're going to notice a dramatic
difference between these exercises and the exercises you have learned. Some of the traditional
ways can be difficult, if not potentially harmful to your body. They can actually increase tension,
instead of releasing it, and be counterproductive to our goals.

Being able to tell the difference between exercises that are good for you and exercises that are
not so good will help you avoid injuries in yoga and other forms of exercise. And by testing these
traditional yoga-based exercises, you can determine for yourself the appropriateness of the
ExTension program.

And as you proceed, ask yourself the following questions: "Do I feel heavy or unbalanced? Do
I feel any strain in my neck or back? Has my breathing become inhibited?" These are some of the
indications that you have lost integrity in the exercise.

LUNGE

The traditional Lunge has you
simply stretching your left
leg out behind you and
looking up at the ceiling,
with your front knee well
forward of its ankle. As you
do it now [Fig.190], notice
how your neck tenses up.
Many people will also

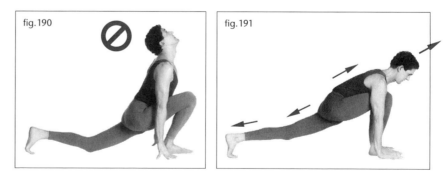

fig.190

fig.191

experience some discomfort in the forward knee. Another common Lunge variation extends the
rear leg with the knee off the floor [Fig.191], dramatically increasing the stretch in the hips, groin,
and thighs. Although I teach this variation to more experienced students, it is not recommended
for beginners.

POSE OF THE CHILD

To test the traditional Pose of the Child, get into position, then place your forehead on the floor [Fig. 192]. Unless you are very supple, you will feel your neck or shoulders tensing almost immediately. If you pay attention, you will also notice that it becomes hard to get a full, deep breath in this position.

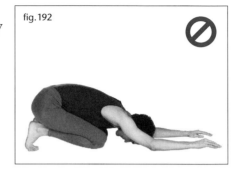

fig. 192

Since the object of the Pose of the Child is to relax, to release tension through extension (especially in the neck, shoulders, and back), and to enhance the transportation of oxygen throughout the body, it makes little sense to place your head down on the floor.

COBRA

In a traditional Cobra, your hands are on the floor beneath or behind your shoulders. You then push up [Fig. 193] and arch your head back as far as you can [Fig. 194]. Straightening your elbows, you push back

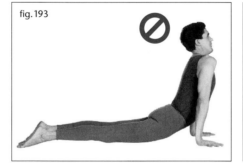

fig. 193

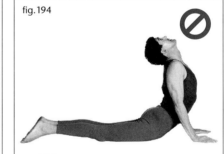

fig. 194

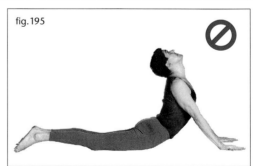

fig. 195

even more [Fig. 195]. Carefully try that now, but don't push to the point of pain in your lower back or neck; just pay attention to what you feel. It may be a compression in your lower back, ranging from mild to severe, a tightness in your neck and shoulders, or fatigue in your neck, back, arms, or wrists. Even if you don't feel pain now as you push back, you'll probably feel your breathing become restricted. And if your head is thrown back, your throat will become overstretched and tight. Try talking with your head thrown back. Is it easy and comfortable? Probably not. All the exercises in this book should be done without strain anywhere, including, as with this exercise, the throat.

DOWNWARD FACING DOG

To do a traditional Downward Facing Dog pose, start on your hands and knees. Then straighten your legs and arms and lift your hips toward the ceiling so that your body forms an inverted "V." Your legs are now locked straight, heels are down on the floor, and your head is dropped below the shoulders.

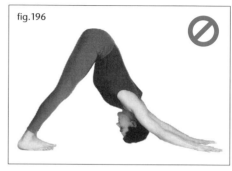

fig.196

The emphasis here is on taking your head and chest close to the floor by dropping your head and pushing your shoulders downward as far as you can toward your feet [Fig.196]. As you carefully try this, feel what happens to your neck, shoulders, or back (and, unless you are very flexible, the tendons behind your knees).

If you could look in a mirror, you would see how awkward it looks. Notice what happens to your breathing. Is it harder to breathe deeply? Does the position hurt? Compared to the ExTension Dog pose, you're doing way too much work here. Less, when done correctly, will always get you more.

TRIANGLE

The traditional Triangle pose, also called a side bend, starts with your feet apart, about three to three and a half feet wide (narrower for short legs, wider for long legs), and parallel. Keeping your shoulders and hips directly parallel with the wall in front of you, bend your torso to your right side and place your right hand down on your right shin. Stretch your left arm up over your head

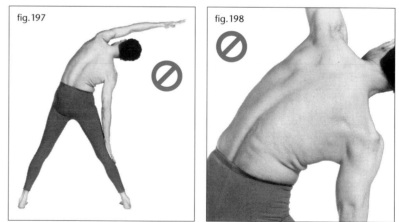

fig.197

fig.198

[Fig.197]. (You might want to keep your abdominal muscles contracted to protect your back.)

While you're bent over sideways, take your hands and feel the flesh around both sides of your waist. The right side probably feels bunched up and contracted, the left side stretching, maybe even overstretching [Fig.198]. More important, can you feel what's happening to your lower back on the right side? Does it feel compressed? The farther down you go, the more you compress the soft tissue structures of the low back.

WARRIOR

You've already tested the Warrior with soft arms (page 132) and discovered that if you don't extend through your arms and hands, the pose feels imbalanced and uncomfortable. The traditional Warrior leaves out many of the details that make it work, and feel better. From the Mountain pose, step wider than you did in the Triangle pose — about four to four and a half feet. Turn your right foot toward the right 90 degrees. Turn your left foot inward to the right about half that amount. Raise your arms out to the side but this time, lean way to the right really extending your right arm [Fig. 199] as you bend your right knee. Hold for a few deep breaths, then come up.

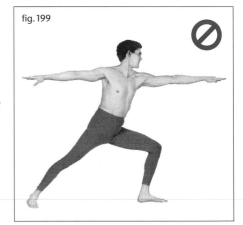

fig. 199

Did you notice how quickly your arms and right leg tired? Did you notice any strain in your right knee as it moved beyond its ankle? You can tell the difference if you immediately follow this traditional variation with the ExTension Warrior (page 130) adhering to the details, especially active arms and proper leg and knee placement.

SHOULDER STAND

Before we test a traditional Shoulder Stand, let's explore an important concept about the ExTension Shoulder Stand by testing the "extension releases tension" theory in another context. Follow the details going up into the posture appropriate for your body type (refer back to pages 140–147). Then allow your legs to go soft by letting go of the action in your feet and legs [Fig. 200]. Keep your legs on the wall but stay up with soft legs for a few breaths. Then bend your knees and slowly roll down.

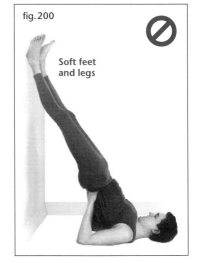

fig. 200

Soft feet and legs

Did you notice how this made your neck and shoulders feel? Did you feel a restriction in your breath or when you talked? Did your eyes feel heavy or protruded? Did it feel as if pressure was building up in your head?

Here's what happened. As your body weight fell downward toward your neck (because of inactive legs and feet), your neck was crushed down into the floor. The rear neck tissues — the muscles, tendons, and ligaments — all overstretched. The structures of your throat were squeezed and compressed, including your larynx (voice box), trachea (windpipe), and carotid arteries of your neck, which are major suppliers of blood to your head. Circulation to your head was reduced and the pressure in your eyes and head increased.

This is why people with glaucoma, detached retina, or high blood pressure should not totally invert their bodies but should stay with the Legs Up the Wall position, keeping their hips on the floor. Legs Up the Wall — along with improved diet — has been known to assist in reducing hypertension.

There are two ways that the traditional Shoulder Stand is practiced: "hanging out" and "pushing up." Both begin by lying flat on the floor, bending your knees and lifting your body up off the floor by simply pulling your legs up toward the ceiling and supporting your hips with your hands.

CAUTION

Do not take your feet to the floor behind your head (sometimes called the Plough). Unless you are very flexible, this puts too much stress on the tissues of your lower back and the back of your neck.

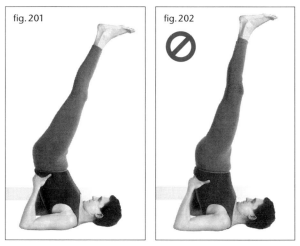

fig. 201   fig. 202

The "hanging out" variation [Fig. 201] is a pretty harmless pose. It doesn't place too much stress on your neck, nor does it significantly inhibit your breath as long as you keep your legs jackknifed at the hips. But as I have said before, it makes little sense to do an inhibiting exercise when you have an ExTension alternative.

The "pushing up" variation [Fig. 202], on the other hand, is not so benign. It squeezes your throat, causes your head to feel heavy and full, compresses your chest, and restricts your breath. It also sometimes causes your eyes to become bloodshot.

Pulling your body up even farther overextends the tendons and ligaments in the back of your neck and compresses your chest and your throat, which restricts your breathing and distorts your speech. When done regularly and consistently over the course of many years, this variation has been known to cause military neck (a reduction or loss of the natural curve of your neck) and even hearing impairment. But even if you can do either of the variations without discomfort, there's really no need to when you have an ExTension alternative.

BRIDGE

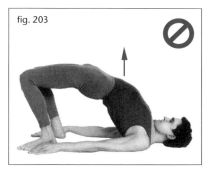

fig. 203

There are several variations of the traditional Bridge pose. In most of them, however, emphasis is placed on arching your back as high as you can. Test that out now. Lie with your back on the floor, knees bent using no head prop, feet flat on the floor and as close to your shoulders as you can get them. Arms remain at your sides. Now, lift your hips as high as you can [Fig. 203]. Try arching your back up higher for just a moment; then come down. How did it feel? Unless you are really flexible, you may have sensed significant compression in your lower back, possible knee pain, and some breathing restriction. But even if you felt no discomfort at all, the traditional Bridge compresses your spine and just as with the Cobra pose, any back compression or pain is inappropriate; even just a little.

Side Twist

The traditional Side Twist is done without jogging your hips, without props, and without active feet and hands [Fig. 204]. Lie on your back with your arms forming a "T," palms up. Bend your knees and keeping your shoulders

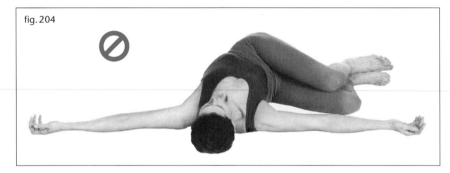

fig. 204

down, roll your knees directly over to your right side and let them down to the floor. You can look straight up or turn your head to look at your left hand. Then bring your knees back up to center, knees bent, feet on the floor, and rest.

Even if it felt okay to you, did you notice if your back seemed at all tense? Was it easy to keep your shoulders down? Did you feel tense anywhere? When you look at Figure 204, notice how the hips are off center from the upper torso. This misalignment places stress on your spinal muscles and does not allow your body to relax fully into the twist. This is supposed to be a relaxing, extending exercise, so tension is counterproductive. Any pain or tightness anywhere in your body sets off a chain reaction in the rest of your body, making it impossible to relax into what's supposed to be a relaxing stretch.

If you immediately follow this with the ExTension Side Twist (see page 156) keeping all the details, especially jogging your hips, and keeping your feet and hands active, you'll notice a big difference between this and the traditional variation.

APPENDIX III

VARIATION FOR HAMSTRING STRETCHING:
WHEN YOU CANNOT FEEL YOUR HAMSTRINGS STRETCH

Do this variation if, in any of the poses or tests in this book, you can't clearly and definitely isolate your hamstring stretch. (It's also a preparation for the ExTension Shoulder Stand.)

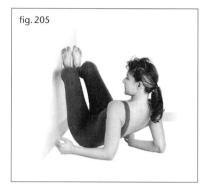

fig. 205

Sit sideways about 12 inches away from a wall [Fig. 205 for tighter people, Fig. 206 for more flexible people]. Lie back and roll your legs up [Fig. 207 for tighter people, Fig. 208 for more flexible people]. With your hand, feel if your tailbone is flat on the floor; if it is, and your back has a natural arch in it, you're in the right position. If your tailbone comes off the floor or if your lower back is flat to the floor, you need to scoot farther away from the wall.

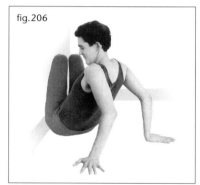

fig. 206

Keep your left leg stretching up the wall but bend your right knee and place your right foot flat on the wall, with the ankle next to your left knee [Fig. 209 for tighter people, Fig. 210 for more flexible people]. Extend your left leg, keeping the knee bent only enough to keep the stretch out of the tendons directly behind the knee. Now fully flex your left foot and extend through the heel. Do you feel an easy stretch in your left hamstring? If so, relax there; if not, scoot your buttocks closer to, or farther from, the wall either to intensify or reduce the stretch.

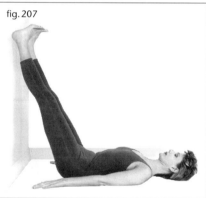

fig. 207

If the stretch is too intense, or you feel it behind your left knee, bend your left leg only enough to release the stretch. The object is to position yourself close enough to the wall so that you can keep your tailbone down and still feel a natural arch in your back and an isolated action in your hamstrings. Hold the stretch for six to twelve long, deep, easy breaths, then switch to the other leg.

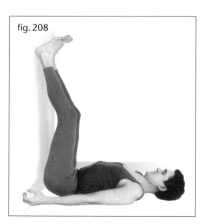

fig. 208

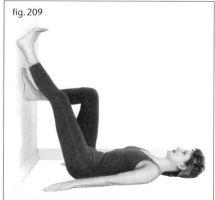

fig. 209

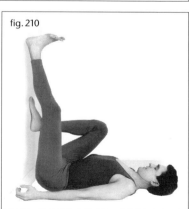

fig. 210

A P P E N D I X   IV

Progressive Relaxation
(In Detail)

FINE-TUNING

A good way to practice is to tape-record your own voice speaking the following progressive relaxation in a slow, soothing voice being sure to pause between "phrases" (where you see the ellipses). Then play it back during your relaxation segment. The words in parentheses are directions, so don't speak them aloud.

You're lying on the floor; your body is in a comfortable position, your hands are softly curled. Feel your body as it lays upon the floor.... Now take a long, deep soft inhalation...then slowly exhale, allowing your exhalation to last longer than your inhalation....

Take another deep, deep inhalation, and let out a long, slow, deep, soft exhalation...one more deep, deep, soft inhalation...then a long, slow, deep exhalation, lasting longer than the inhalation. (Pause 15–20 seconds.)

Now, gently, without becoming aggressive, take a deep inhalation and tense the toes of both your feet. Tighten, tighten, tighten.... Now exhale and let them go....

Move on to your ankles and calves...inhale...tighten, tighten, tighten...and exhale and relax....

Go on to your knees...inhale...tighten the knees, tighten, tighten tighten...exhale and relax....

Bring your awareness to your thighs. Breathe in...tense them up, tense tense, tense, tense...exhale and relax....

Now your hips and buttocks...inhale...tense, tense, tense, tense, tense...exhale...release and relax....

Bring awareness to your belly. Take a deep inhalation...tense the belly, tense, tense, tense...exhale and relax the belly....

Bring awareness to your back. Inhale...tense, tense, tense your back...hold...exhale and relax....

Now your hands and your fingers. Breathe in...make a fist...tight, tight, tight...and exhale and relax. Allow your hands to be very soft. Remember to curl your fingertips....

Bring awareness to your arms, the lower and upper arms...inhale...tense, tense, tense...hold...exhale, and relax....

Bring awareness now to your throat. Inhale...tense your throat...tense, tense, tense...exhale and relax....

Bring awareness now to your face. Inhale and purse, tense, tense your lips...exhale and relax.... Now open your mouth wide...hold...and relax your mouth. Relax your tongue off the palate.

(Begin speaking very slow and gently.) Very gently now, tense and release your eyes.... Tense your eyebrows...hold and release....Tense your forehead and release.... Just relax...relax...relax.... (Pause for 15–20 seconds.)

And now, with every breath you take and with every beat of your heart, relax...relax...relax.

Deeper and deeper...letting go of your body...allow it to sink deeper and deeper into the floor....

Now, I'm going to count from five down to the number one, and with every number that I count, relax deeper...deeper and deeper into the floor.... (Repeat.)

Five, relaxing your entire body.... (Pause ten seconds.)

Four, as you exhale, feel your body sinking even deeper and deeper into the floor.... (Pause ten seconds.)

Three, relaxing your eyes and feeling them sinking deeper and deeper into your head.... (Pause ten seconds.)

Two, allowing your belly to relax and feeling your belly sinking deeper into your body....(Pause ten seconds.)

And...one, completely and totally relaxed. More relaxed than you have been in a long, long, time. Relax. Relax. Relax....(Pause ten seconds.)

Observe how quiet your body is. Should you fall asleep, just remember that that is what you need and it is perfectly all right...to relax...relax...relax....

(After several minutes, begin speaking very softly.) Now, I am going to count from the number one to the number five.... I am going to count from the number one to the number five.... And as I count up, slowly bring your body back to awareness.

(Pause ten seconds between the numbers).

One, slowly bring awareness to your body as it lies upon the floor.

Two, take a gentle but deep breath.

Three, bring feeling back to your body by wiggling your fingers and toes.

Four, begin stretching your arms and your legs.

Five, open your eyes, feeling refreshed and relaxed.

Then, when you are ready, slowly place yourself into any comfortable seated position (elevating your seat with a folded blanket or large book). Take a few moments sitting quietly before standing up and going about the rest of your day feeling relaxed and refreshed.

Appendix V

Who Will Stop the Pain?

Survey results from *Backache Relief,* Times Books / Random House, 1985; paperback: NAL / Signet Books

by Arthur Klein and Dava Sobel

Practitioner	Moderate-to-Dramatic Long-Term Relief (%)	Temporary Relief (%)
Yoga Instructors	96	4
Physiatrists	86	0
Physical Therapists	65	8
Acupuncturists	36	32
Chiropractors	28	28
Osteopathic Physicians	28	15
Neurosurgeons	26	8
Orthopedists	23	9
Family Practitioners	20	14
Massage Therapists	10	63
Neurologists	4	4

The Muscular System

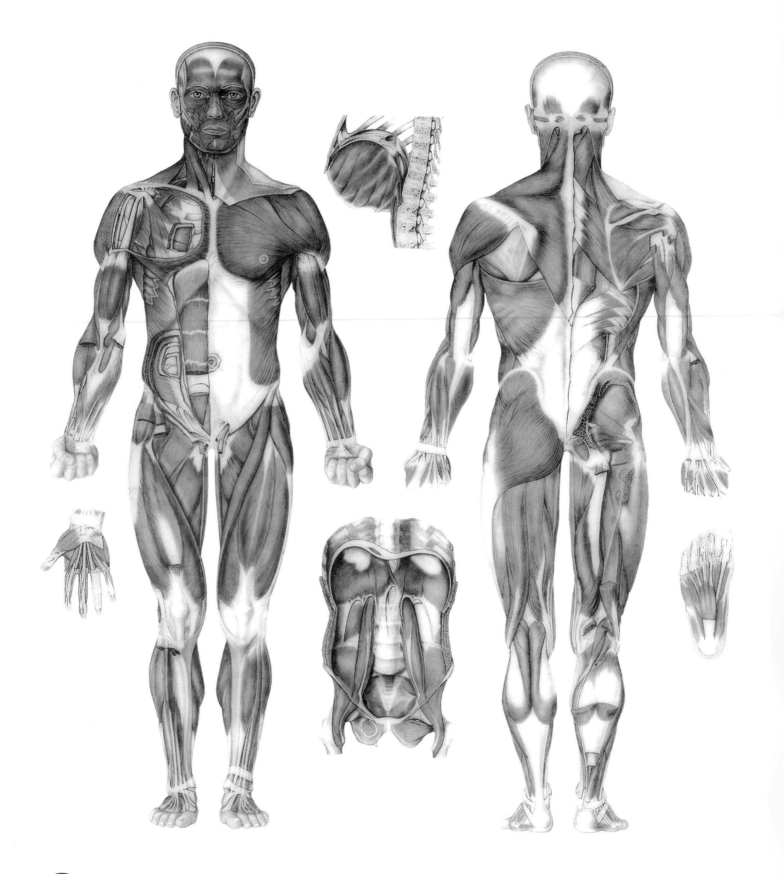

THE SKELETAL SYSTEM

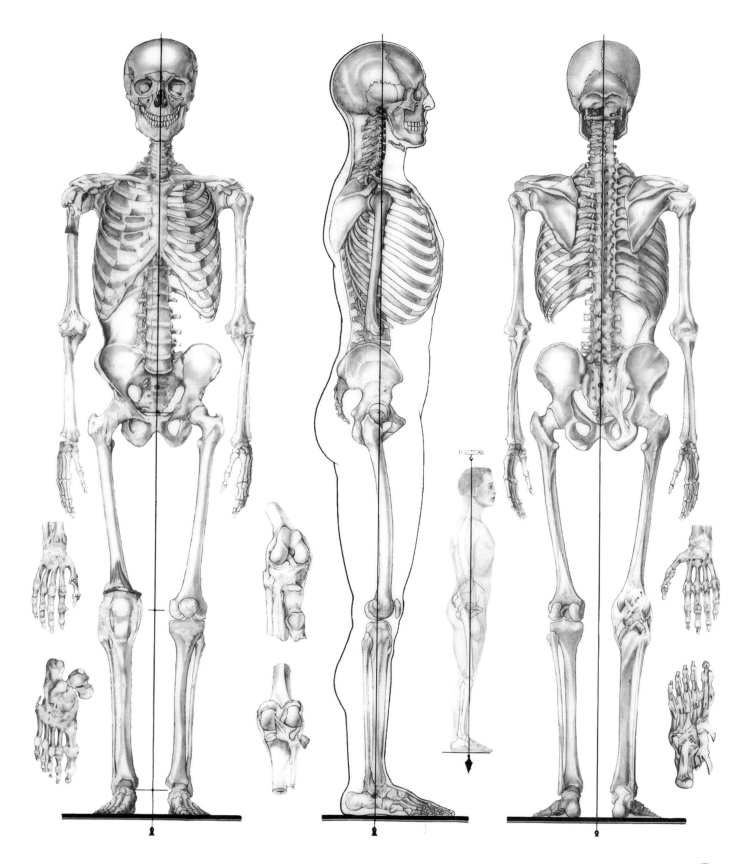

CLEMENTE'S *ANATOMY* SHOWING FASCIA

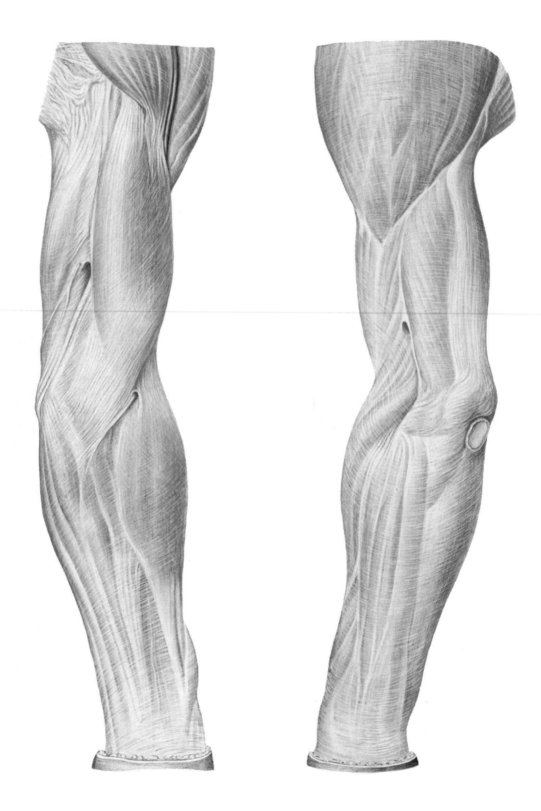

Clemente's *Anatomy* Showing Fascia

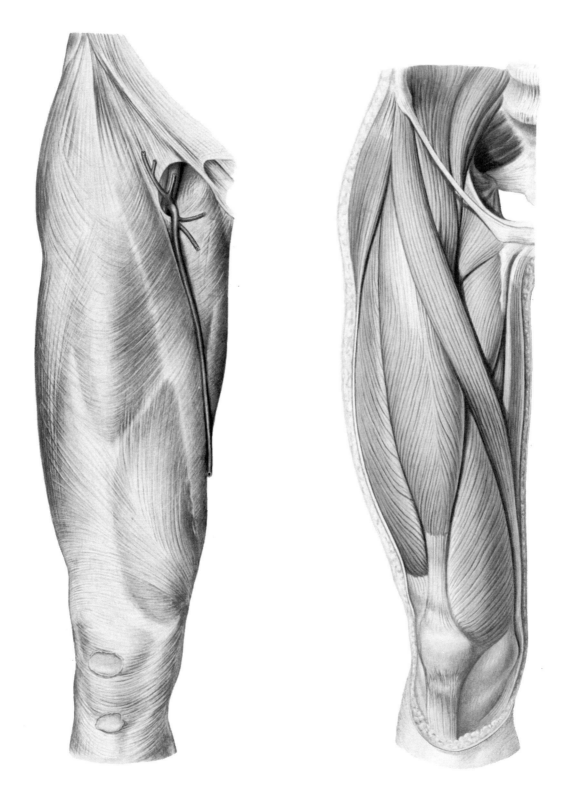

Resources

Carpet samples or remnants can be purchased from almost any carpet dealer.
They often have samples from discontinued lines, and prices are usually low or negotiable.
Some come already bound or they can be bound at an additional cost.

•

To purchase an individual copy or for subscription information, write:
Yoga Journal
2054 University Avenue
Berkeley, CA 94704

•

For information on setting up seminars in your area, write me:
Sam Dworkis
c/o Donald Cleary
Jane Rotrosen Agency
318 East 51 Street
New York, NY 10022